Statistical Approaches in Oncology Clinical Development

Chapman & Hall/CRC Biostatistics Series

RECENTLY PUBLISHED TITLES

Bayesian Methods for Repeated Measures
Lyle D. Broemeling

Modern Adaptive Randomized Clinical Trials: Statistical and Practical Aspects
Oleksandr Sverdlov

Medical Product Safety Evaluation: Biological Models and Statistical Methods
Jie Chen, Joseph Heyse, Tze Leung Lai

Statistical Methods for Survival Trial Design: With Applications to Cancer Clinical Trials Using R
Jianrong Wu

Platform Trials in Drug Development: Umbrella Trials and Basket Trials
Zoran Antonjevic and Robert Beckman

For more information about this series, please visit: https://www.crcpress.com/go/biostats

Statistical Approaches in Oncology Clinical Development

Current Paradigm and Methodological Advancement

Edited by

Satrajit Roychoudhury

and Soumi Lahiri

CRC Press
Taylor & Francis Group
Boca Raton London New York

CRC Press is an imprint of the
Taylor & Francis Group, an **informa** business
A CHAPMAN & HALL BOOK

CRC Press
Taylor & Francis Group
6000 Broken Sound Parkway NW, Suite 300
Boca Raton, FL 33487-2742

Printed on acid-free paper

International Standard Book Number-13: 978-1-4987-7269-3 (Hardback)

Library of Congress Cataloging-in-Publication Data

Names: Roychoudhury, Satrajit, editor. | Lahiri, Soumi, editor.
Title: Statistical approaches in oncology clinical development / [edited by] Satrajit Roychoudhury, Soumi Lahiri.
Description: Boca Raton: Taylor & Francis, 2018. | Includes bibliographical references and index.
Identifiers: LCCN 2018028747 | ISBN 9781498772693 (hardback: alk. paper)
Subjects: | MESH: Neoplasms—drug therapy | Clinical Trials as Topic | Drug Design | Models, Statistical
Classification: LCC RC271.C5 | NLM QZ 267 | DDC 616.99/4061—dc23
LC record available at https://lccn.loc.gov/2018028747

Visit the Taylor & Francis Web site at
http://www.taylorandfrancis.com

and the CRC Press Web site at
http://www.crcpress.com

To my beloved family and in loving memory of my mother

Satrajit Roychoudhury

Contents

Contents

Preface

Oncology is a rapidly developing area in medical science. A significant investment in terms of costs, resources, and time is required for oncology drug development. Therefore, an understanding of the challenges in each phase is critical for a successful drug launch. The purpose of this book is to provide an overview and state-of-the-art statistical solutions to some of these challenges commonly observed during planning, conducting, and reporting of cancer trials. Well-known and experienced statisticians from the pharmaceutical industry, academia, and US Food and Drug Administration (FDA) have contributed to writing a chapter each in this book. The book includes many examples of real-life cancer trials to elaborate the utility of modern statistical methodologies. In addition, the book includes relevant statistical codes to facilitate practical implementation. The topics covered are:

- General overview of statistical approaches in oncology clinical development (Chapter 1)
- Design and analysis of early phase cancer trials (Chapter 2)
- Role of exposure–response analysis (Chapter 3)
- Statistical methods in evaluating predictive biomarker in cancer (Chapter 4)
- Design consideration in Phase II trials (Chapter 5)
- Role of precision medicine and associated challenges in oncology drug development (Chapter 6)
- Use of adaptive design in oncology confirmatory trials (Chapter 7)
- Methodologies for safety monitoring and analysis in oncology trials (Chapter 8)
- Analysis and reporting of the quality-of-life data (Chapter 9)
- Evolving regulatory pathways on statistical considerations in oncology clinical trials (Chapter 10)

Many of these topics are less understood and pose challenges in the design and analysis of cancer trials. Many of the methodologies discussed in this book have applications in other therapeutic areas. The primary audience of this book will be statisticians with postgraduate training and working on cancer trials in the pharmaceutical industry, academia, and regulatory agencies. Although it is not intended as a textbook, practitioners may find this book useful as a supplementary material. Moreover, key opinion leaders and strategy makers in oncology will find this book useful.

Acknowledgment

We would like to thank the reviewers for their valuable inputs, which have helped us to improve the overall quality of the book. We personally thank Dr. Beat Neuenschwander, Novartis Pharma AG, Basel, Switzerland; Dr. Pulak Ghosh, Indian Institute of Management, Bangalore, India; and Dr. Paul Gallo, Novartis Pharmaceutical Company, East Hanover, New Jersey, for numerous scientific discussions regarding the design and analysis of cancer trials. A special thanks to Dr. Kannan Natarajan, Dr. Demissie Alemayehu, and Dr. Neal Thomas from Pfizer Inc. for the management support. Last but not least, we would like to thank CRC Acquisition Editor John Kimmel for his support and work in this book publishing project.

Satrajit Roychoudhury
Senior Director, Pfizer Inc.

Soumi Lahiri
Independent Statistical Professional

Acknowledgment

Editors

Satrajit Roychoudhury is a Senior Director and a member of the Statistical Research and Innovation group at Pfizer Inc. Prior to joining, he was a member of the Statistical Methodology and Consulting Group in Novartis. He has 11 years of extensive experience in working with different phases of clinical trials. His area of research includes early phase oncology trials, survival analysis, model-informed drug development, and use of Bayesian methods in clinical trials. He is the industry co-chair for the ASA Biopharmaceutical Section Regulatory-Industry Workshop and has provided statistical training in major conferences including the Joint Statistical Meetings, ASA Biopharmaceutical Section Regulatory-Industry Workshop, and ICSA Applied Statistics Symposium.

Soumi Lahiri has 12 years of extensive experience in working in different therapeutic areas. She is the former Director of Biostatistics in Clinical Oncology, GlaxoSmithKline. She has also worked in the oncology division of Novartis Pharmaceutical Company for 2 years. She is an active member of the ASA Biopharmaceutical section and former chair of the membership committee.

Contributors

Ohad Amit
Clinical Statistics
GlaxoSmithKline
Collegeville, Pennsylvania

Arunava Chakravartty
Biostatistics and Pharmacometrics
Novartis Pharmaceuticals
Company
East Hanover, New Jersey

Yi-Lin Chiu
Biometrics
AbbVie Inc.
Chicago, Illinois

Diane Fairclough
Colorado School of Public Health
Denver, Colorado

Jared C. Foster
Biostatistics Branch
National Cancer Institute
Rockville, Maryland

Balakrishna S. Hosmane
AbbVie Inc.
Chicago, Illinois

Anastasia Ivanova
Department of Biostatistics
University of North Carolina at
Chapel Hill
Chapel Hill, North Carolina

Qi Jiang
Biometrics
Seattle Genetics
Bothell, Washington

Jennifer Le-Rademacher
Division of Biomedical Statistics and
Informatics
Mayo Clinic
Rochester, New York

Sumithra J. Mandrekar
Division of Biomedical Statistics and
Informatics
Mayo Clinic
Rochester, New York

Olga Marchenko
Department of Biostatistics
Bayer Pharmaceutical
Whippany, New Jersey

Pabak Mukhopadhyay
Biostatistics and Pharmacometrics
Novartis Pharmaceuticals Company
East Hanover, New Jersey

Satrajit Roychoudhury
Statistical Research and Innovation
Pfizer Inc.
New York, New York

Jaya Satgopan
Department of Biostatistics and
Epidemiology
Memorial Sloan Kettering Cancer
Center
New York, New York

Sanjay S. Shete
Department of Biostatistics
The University of Texas MD
Anderson Cancer Center
Houston, Texas

Rajeshwari Sridhara
Division of Biostatistics
Center for Drug Evaluation and Research
U.S. Federal Drug Administration
Silver Spring, Maryland

Rajesh Talluri
Data Sciences
The University of Mississippi Medical Center
Jackson, Mississippi

Simon Wandel
Statistical Research and Consulting
Novartis Pharma AG
Basel, Switzerland

Richard C. Zink
TARGET PharmaSolutions
University of North Carolina at Chapel Hill
Chapel Hill, North Carolina

1

Introduction

Ohad Amit
GlaxoSmithKline

In 2010, the I-SPY2 trial [1] was launched as an innovative collaboration across five pharmaceutical companies in a phase 2 breast cancer trial. The benefits of this collaborative approach, which significantly reduces the cost, time, and number of subjects required for efficiently bringing new drug therapies to patients, embodies the culmination of much of the innovation in statistical methodology that has characterized oncology drug development in recent years.

Unlike other disease areas, the statistical methodology supporting oncology drug development has long been specialized and has evolved independently of other clinical trial methodologies. The unmet need and urgency underpinning oncology drug development have put many new innovations in statistical methodology front and center.

Fundamentally, the endpoints used to evaluate new therapeutics in oncology have not changed over the last 30 years. Tumor shrinkage, disease progression, and overall survival (OS) remain the mainstays for evaluating the efficacy of new treatments in phase 2 and phase 3 trials. These endpoints confer a readily interpretable result for researchers in a great majority of trials and have been at the core of significant advances in treatment over the last few years. But there is fertile ground to move beyond these traditional modalities. The emergence of more sophisticated imaging modalities and new biomarkers resulting from a more granular understanding of cancer at the molecular level has created tremendous opportunities to further expedite the development of new cancer therapeutics. These new markers can be predictive, defining an enriched population more likely to benefit from treatment, or can be used to evaluate the efficacy of new treatments.

Despite the promises held by these new endpoints, single-arm trials with endpoints based on tumor shrinkage remain the mainstay of phase 2 development in oncology. Such trials rely on the use of historical controls to draw inferences based on well-established response criteria, such as Response evaluation criteria in solid tumors (RECIST) [2]. Such trials are well-placed to incorporate Bayesian methods, and methods have been developed to continuously monitor the data emerging from these trials in a Bayesian decision framework. In many situations, single-arm trials have provided an efficient framework for speeding the approval of new agents. This is particularly true of agents with transformational efficacy where response rates are observed significantly in excess of what one might expect, with last line therapy where few treatment options are available. However, in many other settings, single-arm trials remain difficult to interpret. For agents whose activity is more cytostatic in nature, single-arm trials have been designed with the aim of evaluating efficacy based on the comparison of a time-to-event endpoint relative to historical control. Unlike tumor shrinkage, with time-to-event endpoints in such a trial, there is inherent difficulty in differentiating between the natural history of disease and treatment efficacy. Similarly, with combination agents studied in a single-arm trial, there are inherent challenges in differentiating monotherapy activity from combination efficacy in the absence of a control arm. In both these situations, randomized trials are typically needed. Randomized trials are longer, larger, and more expensive than single-arm trials. There is an opportunity and a clear need to develop new, more efficient designs in these situations.

Unlike in phase 2, progression free survival (PFS) and overall survival (OS) remain the mainstays in phase 3 trials. As more and more effective therapies become available across many tumor types, OS is becoming an increasingly difficult endpoint to study. Long OS times and confounding of results from effective post-progression therapies have greatly complicated the ability to design trials with OS as a primary objective. However, in later line settings or histologies where survival times are shorter, there is a stronger rationale for using OS as a primary endpoint. A key challenge in designing trials with an OS endpoint in later lines for later lines of treatment centers around whether subjects randomized to the control arm should be allowed to crossover to the experimental arm at the time of progression. Many cogent ethical arguments have been made for and against allowing such crossover. What remains indisputable, however, is that allowing crossover will complicate and confound the ability to estimate an unbiased treatment effect with respect to OS. Several statistical methods have been developed over the last few years to provide for more accurate estimates of the treatment effect on OS in the presence of potentially confounding post-progression therapies.

With complications in the evaluation of OS, PFS has rapidly gained traction in many settings as a key endpoint in phase 3 evaluation. Much has been written in the literature over the last few years about the methodological challenges in both the assessment and statistical analysis of PFS. At the core of this discussion is a debate around whether a treatment effect on PFS represents clinical benefit in and of itself or whether PFS is a surrogate for OS. Demonstrating the surrogacy of PFS has been accomplished in some histologies but in general has remained challenging. There has been growing acceptance of the PFS as an endpoint which measures the clinical benefit directly. A large treatment effect in terms of PFS strengthens the argument of clinical benefit. However, many methodologic challenges remain. These include optimizing the interval for assessment and scanning frequency, handling dropouts and missing data, and the need and value of a blinded central independent review. The recent introduction of new immuno-oncology therapies has also created new challenges in the evaluation of PFS.

The endpoints and associated trial designs in oncology have been responsible for many successful development programs in oncology, but often times registration has not been with the optimal dose regimen. Dose selection remains a critical challenge in the development of new oncology therapeutics. Unfortunately, the traditional paradigm developed for cytotoxic drugs of identifying the maximum tolerated dose (MTD) and subsequent p2 and 3 doses based on dose-limiting toxicities remains entrenched as a key feature of early development in many of the oncology programs. Over the last few years, this approach has led to several undesirable outcomes, including multiple sponsors having to initiate post-marketing commitments to further refine the dosing regimen. The oncology literature is rich with various dose escalation schemes for identifying the MTD. Many of these methods incorporate statistical modeling and formal use of historical data via Bayesian methods. There is hopefully little controversy in the notion that statistical modeling and Bayesian methods should be at the core of any dose-selection strategy. The current opportunity is to parlay these methods into more robust p2 trial designs that allow for a more informed evaluation and differentiation of doses based on risk and benefit.

In 2015, the United States government launched the precision medicine initiative, validating many of the novel concepts incorporated into the I-SPY2 trial 5 years earlier. The mission of this initiative is *"To enable a new era of medicine through research, technology, and policies that empower patients, researchers, and providers to work together toward development of individualized care."* For many years now oncology has been at the forefront of precision medicine, with many examples now of targeted therapies approved based on the individual molecular and genetic profile of the tumor. The mission of the precision medicine initiative has the potential to open tremendous opportunities for statistical innovation in oncology. The evaluation of medicines in the context of precision medicines requires a new approach to trial design in early and late phases of drug development. It also necessitates consideration of companion diagnostics, and there are many other nontraditional statistical methods that could be considered. Such initiatives leave oncology and its researchers poised to break down the doors and enter a new and exciting era of drug development, an era that will undoubtedly be characterized by many bold statistical innovations.

The following chapters present a comprehensive review of many of the important statistical aspects of oncology drug development, many of which directly address the challenges described earlier. The first five chapters focus on early development including phase 1 and phase 2 trials, model-based approaches, and biomarker-based approaches. The remaining chapters focus on later phase development including phase 3 trials, quality of life, risk benefit, and regulatory challenges.

We hope this book proves useful and provides a comprehensive treatment for all relevant statistical issues in oncology.

References

1. Barker, A., Sigman, C., Kelloff, G., Hylton, N., Berry, D., and Esserman, L. (2009), I-SPY 2: An adaptive breast cancer trial design in the setting of neoadjuvant chemotherapy. *Clinical Pharmacology & Therapeutics*, 86: 97–100.
2. Eisenhauer, E.A., Therasse, P., Bogaerts, J., Schwartz, L.H., Sargent, D., Ford, R., Dancey, J., Arbuck, S., Gwyther, S., Mooney, M., Rubinstein, L., Shankar, L., Dodd, L., Kaplan, R., Lacombe, D., Verweij, J. (2009), New response evaluation criteria in solid tumours: Revised RECIST guideline (version 1.1). *European Journal of Cancer*, 45(2): 228–247.

2

Statistical Considerations in Phase I Oncology Trials

Simon Wandel
Novartis Pharma AG

Satrajit Roychoudhury
Pfizer Inc.

CONTENTS

2.1 Introduction

Phase I trials in oncology aim at identifying a maximum tolerated dose (MTD) or a recommended phase II dose (RP2D) of a new anticancer therapy. An important difference between phase I trials in oncology and first-in-human (FIH) studies in other therapeutic areas is the study population—outside oncology, healthy volunteers are studied, whereas in oncology, terminally ill patients are enrolled. This difference originates from the fact that most oncology drugs can cause (eventually severe) side effects and it would be unethical to expose healthy volunteers to these drugs. However, they can be the last option for patients with end-stage, non-treatable cancer, who may be willing to accept some level of toxicity. The dilemma when conducting oncology phase I studies is, therefore, the following—escalation should happen quickly to reach a potentially efficacious dose, while overly aggressive dose increments could expose patients to unacceptable toxicities. A good phase I study design needs to address this dilemma prospectively, and we will discuss the corresponding challenges and potential solutions in Section 2.2.

Another challenge during dose escalation is the limited number of patients who are evaluated at the most interesting dose, that is, the MTD/RP2D. Typically, only one or two cohorts (around 6 to 12 patients) are studied at this dose. Furthermore, the patient population is often heterogeneous, which makes it difficult to interpret potential efficacy signals. Therefore, most phase I studies enter an expansion phase once the MTD/RP2D is declared, during which more patients are investigated. In recent years, the expansion phase has attracted particular interest in the phase I community (Manji et al., 2013), and it has proven useful in the early development of oncology drugs. Especially for targeted therapies, it can be interesting to collect data in a homogeneous population during expansion and therefore provide more reliable and relevant evidence for decision-making. The expansion phase offers a variety of options to make phase I studies even more valuable for drug development, yet it often remains undiscussed in the literature. Therefore, the entire Section 2.3 is dedicated to this topic. Finally, we will end the chapter with some conclusions, where we will reflect on the subject and put it into a broader perspective.

2.2 Dose Escalation in Phase I Studies

In the previous section, we introduced the main dilemma when conducting phase I studies—one should quickly escalate the dose, while not exposing patients to unacceptable toxicities. This leads to the following question: What constitutes an unacceptable toxicity? In order to answer it, the concept of the dose-limiting toxicity (DLT) has been introduced. Dose-limiting toxicities are severe toxicities that, if occurring too frequently, quantify a dose as being unacceptable to patients. In this sense, DLTs guide the determination of the MTD/RP2D (Eisenhauer, Twelves, & Buyse, 2006). Importantly, however, there is no unique definition of DLTs (Le Tourneau et al., 2011), and the exact definition, which is compound-specific, needs to be provided in the study protocol. Despite a clear definition of DLTs, there are a few other guiding principles that should be followed when planning phase I trials. The principles can be summarized as follows:

1. Clear definition of the adverse events constituting a DLT
2. Careful choice of the first (starting) dose based on preclinical information
3. Sequential enrollment of patients in cohorts of size 3–6
4. Sufficient safety follow-up (typically at least 1 cycle) for each patient
5. Limit on the maximal dose increment—typically 100% for small molecules.

Of course, some flexibility with respect to these principles is allowed. For example, other cohort sizes (1–3 patients) or larger dose increments (e.g., threefold for immune therapies or biologics) may be used. However, these choices should always have a good rational and it should be clear that they do not expose patients to unnecessary risks, in order to comply with the overarching goal of *safety first*!

2.2.1 Operational Aspects

The typical course of a phase I trial follows from the previous principles—the first cohort of patients is enrolled at the starting dose, and after their safety data is available, a decision is made for the dose of the next cohort, which can be the same, lower, or higher dose. This procedure is repeated until the MTD/RP2D is reached or the trial is stopped, for example, because no dose is considered acceptable.

When conducting a phase I trial, one of the most important operational tasks is the dose-escalation meeting. In this meeting, the attendees decide on the dose for the next cohort based on the available evidence and the approach used for the escalation. Notably, during the course of the study, multiple dose-escalation meetings are conducted, since more than one dose escalation typically happens. The data presented during the dose-escalation meeting usually consist of the DLT information for each patient, a summary of the adverse events observed in the trial, pharmacokinetic (PK), pharmacodynamic, and efficacy information. Additionally, the eligible doses for the next cohort as per the dose-escalation approach are presented. This meeting, therefore, requires a number of participants, including the investigators, the physician and statistician of the sponsor, and eventually other experts such as pharmacokineticists and biomarker specialists.

The decision on the dose for the next cohort is often driven by a mix of quantitative and qualitative assessments. While quantitative assessments, such as the DLT rate by dose, are needed to define the range of eligible doses, qualitative assessments, such as the investigators' considerations of an individual patient profile, help to decide on the actual next dose. Therefore, it is the totality of the evidence that ultimately leads to the dose-escalation decision.

One can imagine that a good preparation of the dose-escalation meeting is critical. Even though we could conduct a dose-escalation meeting immediately after the last patient in the cohort had reached the required follow-up (or had experienced a DLT), this is difficult in practice. It often requires substantial time to prepare the data and additional complexities such as shipping samples to laboratories and awaiting their analysis need to be accounted for. Furthermore, dose-escalation meetings need to be well documented, which includes the write-up of the meeting minutes. Good study management and planning ahead of time is therefore critical to ensure a smooth dose escalation.

The actual conduct of dose-escalation meetings may differ between studies. Therefore, it is important that the dose-escalation process is well described in the study protocol, especially since it is the most critical part in a phase I trial. An example of such a description can be found in (Radona, Lin, Robson, Dai, Hailman, & Chica, 2010), which may serve as a reference when developing a phase I protocol.

2.2.2 Statistical Aspects

The primary endpoint of dose escalation studies, the DLT rate, is described by a binary variable, the occurrence of DLT (yes/no). At each tested dose d, the available data are the number of patients with DLT r_d out of the total number of patients n_d; however, the underlying, unknown DLT rate π_d is the quantity of interest. As statisticians, we want to estimate (or model) π_d and reflect the uncertainty associated with it. Nevertheless, algorithmic designs, such as the 3+3 (Storer, 1989) completely ignore π_d and simply apply a strict rule based on r_d and n_d. Even though these designs are clearly inferior to statistical, model-based approaches (Jaki, Clive, & Weir, 2013; Nie et al., 2016), it is important to understand that the majority of phase I practitioners still use them (Le Tourneau, Lee, & Siu, 2009; Riviere, Le Tourneau, Paoletti, Dubois, & Zohar, 2015). This can sometimes cause unanticipated questions by investigational review boards which may be unfamiliar with model-based approaches. For a more extensive discussion of the topic, we refer to (Neuenschwander, Matano, Tang, Roychoudhury, Wandel, & Bailey, 2014).

Turning toward a statistical perspective, we are interested in the probabilistic (Bayesian) inference on π_d, which can be classified according to the following three categories:

- $\pi_d \in [0, 0.16)$: underdosing
- $\pi_d \in [0.16, 0.33)$: targeted toxicity
- $\pi_d \in [0.33, 1.00]$: overdosing

This commonly accepted classification allows us to meet the requirement to treat patients at potentially efficacious, yet not overly toxic doses (see Section 2.1) as follows—we aim to find doses with high probability in the targeted toxicity interval, while controlling the probability of overdosing. The latter is known as the concept of escalation with overdose control and was introduced by Babb, Rogatko, & Zacks in 1998. According to this concept, the threshold to judge whether the probability of overdosing is still acceptable or not for the next dose is 25%, indicating that only doses with $P(\pi_d \in [0.33, 1.00]) < 0.25$ are eligible for escalation.

Despite this binding rule, we want to further quantify π_d and the associated uncertainty. In our phase I trials, we therefore graphically present point estimates (mean or median), 95% intervals, and the interval probabilities for all of the above categories. This has proven useful especially in communication with non-statisticians and will be illustrated in the case study in Section 2.2.6.

When using a statistical approach for dose escalation, we need to assess its properties and include them in the protocol. In our experience, two different metrics are useful and should be investigated—operating characteristics and data scenarios. Operating characteristics describe the long-term behavior of the design under various assumed true dose-toxicity relationships. They are used, for example, to assess the targeting rate, which is the probability to select a dose as MTD with true DLT rate in $[0.16, 0.33)$, given a true dose-toxicity relationship. On the other hand, data scenarios are used to assess hypothetical on-study situations. These can be helpful for discussions with clinical colleagues, but also provide assurance that the inference is reasonable and does not allow, for example, too aggressive escalation. An extensive discussion of both metrics is given in (Neuenschwander, Matano, Tang, Roychoudhury, Wandel, & Bailey, 2014) and an example can be found in (Radona, Lin, Robson, Dai, Hailman, & Chica, 2010).

2.2.3 Logistic Model for Single-Agent Escalation

The logistic model for single-agent escalation describing the dose-toxicity relationship is defined as follows. We use the binomial likelihood to model the DLT data at each dose, that is,

$$r_d \sim \text{Binomial}(n_d, \pi_d). \tag{2.1}$$

Since we consider a single-agent escalation, there is only one variable required for the dose d, and we use the logistic model (Neuenschwander,

Branson, & Gsponer, 2008; Neuenschwander, Matano, Tang, Roychoudhury, Wandel, & Bailey, 2014) for the dose-toxicity relationship

$$\text{logit}(\pi_d) = \log(\alpha) + \beta \log(d/d^*). \tag{2.2}$$

Here, d^* is an arbitrary scaling dose, usually chosen as the anticipated MTD. This model is monotone in dose, implies $\pi_d \to 0$ when $d \to 0$ and has the following interpretation of its parameters (Neuenschwander, Matano, Tang, Roychoudhury, Wandel, & Bailey, 2014):

- α is the odds of DLT at dose d^*
- β is the increase in the log-odds of a DLT by a unit increase in log-dose

For example, when $\log(\alpha) = \text{logit}(1/3)$ and $\beta = 0$, this yields $\pi_{d^*} = 1/3$, and doubling the dose will increase the odds of a DLT by the factor 2.

The prior distributions for $\log(\alpha), \log(\beta)$ are chosen as bivariate normal, that is,

$$\begin{pmatrix} \log(\alpha) \\ \log(\beta) \end{pmatrix} \sim BVN\left(\begin{pmatrix} m_1 \\ m_2 \end{pmatrix}, \begin{pmatrix} s_1^2 & cor \cdot s_1 s_2 \\ cor \cdot s_1 s_2 & s_2^2 \end{pmatrix}\right). \tag{2.3}$$

As for any Bayesian model, the specification of the prior distribution is important. If clinical data on the compound are available, they can be incorporated into the prior distribution. This case will be discussed in the next section. If no clinical data are available, preclinical information can be used to specify a weakly informative prior distribution. In this situation, we recommend a simple approach, setting the prior means to plausible values, but allowing for considerable uncertainty. The latter is achieved with $s_1 = 2$, $s_2 = 1$, $cor = 0$, which covers a wide range of values (Neuenschwander, Matano, Tang, Roychoudhury, Wandel, & Bailey, 2014). Alternatively, a more involved derivation of a weakly informative prior based on minimally informative unimodal Beta distributions and a stochastic optimization could be used (Neuenschwander, Branson, M., & Gsponer, 2008). However, results will typically be similar to the simpler, less time-consuming approach.

In addition to π_d, a quantity that has proven useful for risk communication is the predictive number of DLTs, r_d, in n_d patients to be enrolled in the next cohort at dose d. The predictive distribution is given by

$$P(r_d \mid n_d) = \int \text{Binomial}(n_d, \pi_d) f(\pi_d \mid \text{Data}) d\pi_d \tag{2.4}$$

When communicating the risk of DLTs at the next dose, it can be useful to present this predictive distribution in addition to the posterior summaries of π_d. While it can be difficult for study teams to directly translate π_d into the risk for patients in the next cohort, it is straightforward to interpret the predicted number of DLTs, which may contribute to better-informed decision-making.

2.2.4 Meta-Analytic-Combined Model for Single-Agent Escalation with Co-Data

When relevant clinical data are available, we would like to incorporate them in the prior distribution. Various approaches on how to do so have been described in the literature; for an overview, see (Wandel, Schmidli, & Neuenschwander, 2016). All approaches have in common that they relate the existing data to the new data, in one way or another.

For our trials, we use the meta-analytic-predictive (MAP) or the meta-analytic-combined (MAC) approach to incorporate existing data. The MAP prior for the parameter in the new study is the predictive distribution obtained from a meta-analysis of the existing data. It is particularly useful for the following reasons:

- It fully accounts for between-trial heterogeneity.
- There is a limit to the maximum amount of information that can be borrowed from the existing data; this limit is given by the ratio of the within-trial to the between-trial variance (Neuenschwander, Capkun-Niggli, Branson, & Spiegelhalter, 2010).

A challenge with the MAP approach is that it has no closed form solution; we therefore need to approximate it by a mixture of parametric distributions (Schmidli, Gsteiger, Roychoudhury, O'Hagan, Spiegelhalter, & Neuenschwander, 2014). Additionally, the study-external data (i.e., co-data) may change, for example, when coming from ongoing trials; this can cause operational challenges when using the MAP approach. In this situation, we prefer the MAC approach. Importantly, however, whether we use the MAP or the MAC approach is irrelevant; they give identical results (Schmidli, Gsteiger, Roychoudhury, O'Hagan, Spiegelhalter, & Neuenschwander, 2014). Our preference for the MAC approach in the examples presented is therefore purely due to the desire for technical (and operational) simplicity.

Assuming data from $j = 1,\ldots,J$ existing and a new trial *, the MAC model is given by

$$r_{d,j} \sim \text{Binomial}\left(n_{d,j}, \pi_{d,j}\right)$$

$$r_{d,\star} \sim \text{Binomial}\left(n_{d,\star}, \pi_{d,\star}\right)$$

$$\text{logit}\left(\pi_{d,j}\right) = \log\left(\alpha_j\right) + \beta_j \log\left(d/d^\star\right)$$

$$\text{logit}\left(\pi_{d,\star}\right) = \log\left(\alpha_\star\right) + \beta_\star \log\left(d/d^\star\right)$$

$$\begin{pmatrix} \log(\alpha_j) \\ \log(\beta_j) \end{pmatrix} \sim BVN\left(\begin{pmatrix} \mu_1 \\ \mu_2 \end{pmatrix}, \begin{pmatrix} \tau_1^2 & \rho\tau_1\tau_2 \\ \rho\tau_1\tau_2 & \tau_2^2 \end{pmatrix}\right)$$

$$\begin{pmatrix} \log(\alpha_\star) \\ \log(\beta_\star) \end{pmatrix} \sim BVN\left(\begin{pmatrix} \mu_1 \\ \mu_2 \end{pmatrix}, \begin{pmatrix} \tau_1^2 & \rho\tau_1\tau_2 \\ \rho\tau_1\tau_2 & \tau_2^2 \end{pmatrix}\right)$$

Here, the data from all trials, that is, the J existing *and* the new trial (*) are used. The latter is important; if we would only use the data of the J existing trials, we would get the predictive distribution for $\log(\alpha_\star), \log(\beta_\star)$, that is, the MAP prior. We would then need to approximate it and specify it as a prior distribution to perform the analysis for the actual study. As mentioned before, this will result in exactly the same inference for the actual study as the MAC model that uses all data simultaneously.

The MAC model has five parameters for which we need to specify prior distributions—the means μ_1, μ_2, the standard deviations τ_1, τ_2, and the correlation ρ. In most cases, the following specifications may be appropriate:

$$\mu_1 \sim N\left(m_{\mu_1}, s_{\mu_1}^2\right)$$

$$\mu_2 \sim N\left(m_{\mu_2}, s_{\mu_2}^2\right)$$

$$\tau_1 \sim LN\left(m_{\tau_1}, s_{\tau_1}^2\right)$$

$$\tau_2 \sim LN\left(m_{\tau_2}, s_{\tau_2}^2\right)$$

$$\rho \sim Unif(-1,1)$$

where $x \sim LN(m, s^2)$ denotes the log-normal distribution, that is, $\log(x) \sim N(m, s^2)$. In the absence of additional information, default weakly informative priors for μ_1, μ_2 may be specified as $m_{\mu_1} = \text{logit}(m_{d^*}), s_{\mu_1} = 2$ and $m_{\mu_2} = \log(m_{\text{slope}}), s_{\mu_2} = 1$, with m_{d^*} the anticipated mean DLT rate at d^* and m_{slope} the anticipated slope. For the between-trial standard deviations τ_1, τ_2, the similarities of the different studies need to be considered; proposed values depending on the degree of similarity (Neuenschwander, Matano, Tang, Roychoudhury, Wandel, & Bailey, 2014) can be found in Table 2.1. s_{τ_1} and $s_{\tau 2}$ are then used to reflect the uncertainty associated with the similarity. For example, if moderate between-trial heterogeneity is plausible, yet we wish the 95% interval to cover small to substantial values, the following priors will be used:

$$\tau_1 \sim \text{LN}\left(\log(0.25), (\log(2)/1.96)^2\right)$$

$$\tau_2 \sim \text{LN}\left(\log(0.125), (\log(2)/1.96)^2\right)$$

TABLE 2.1

Classification of Between-Trial Heterogeneity

Degree of Between-Trial Heterogeneity	τ_1	τ_2
Small	0.125	0.0625
Moderate	0.250	0.125
Substantial	0.500	0.250
Large	1.000	0.500

For a more extensive discussion of priors for the between-trial heterogeneity, we refer to a general discussion in (Friede, Röver, Wandel, & Neuenschwander, 2016a) and (Friede, Röver, Wandel, & Neuenschwander, 2016b).

2.2.5 Assessing Effective Sample Size

When borrowing information from co-data (e.g., via the MAC approach), it is important to understand how much additional information one brings into the analysis. In order to do so, a quantity known as (prior) effective sample size (*ESS*) is used. The *ESS* can be interpreted as the number of patients that would be needed to enroll in the study to obtain the same amount of information leveraged from study-external data. However, calculation of the *ESS* can be difficult, since for many situations, there is no direct (analytical) solution for it. Several approximations have been proposed, including the variance ratio approach (Neuenschwander, Capkun-Niggli, Branson, & Spiegelhalter, 2010), but also more involved methods (Morita, Thall, & Müller, 2008, 2012). A simple approach to derive the *ESS* is to approximate the distribution of the parameter of interest by a parametric distribution for which the *ESS* can be calculated directly. For example, the posterior (or prior) distribution of the DLT rate at a given dose (π_d) can be approximated by a *Beta*(a, b) distribution, for which it is known that $ESS = a + b$. The approximation itself is straightforward, assuming that the posterior mean $\left(m_{\pi_d}\right)$ and standard deviation $\left(s_{\pi_d}\right)$ of π_d are known. In that case, we obtain

$$ESS = \frac{m_{\pi_d}\left(1 - m_{\pi_d}\right)}{s_{\pi_d}^2} - 1. \tag{2.5}$$

We will use this approach in the case study to derive the *ESS*.

2.2.6 Case Study: Ceritinib for Non–Small Cell Lung Cancer

To illustrate the concepts and model introduced before, we now discuss the two phase I studies of ceritinib (LDK378, Novartis Pharmaceuticals). Ceritinib was developed as a targeted anticancer therapy against the anaplastic lymphoma kinase (*ALK*) gene (Shaw et al., 2014). When ceritinib was available for clinical development, another potent ALK inhibitor, crizotinib, was already in late clinical development (Shaw et al., 2013) with promising phase I data (Kwak et al., 2010). However, in preclinical experiments, ceritinib showed much higher potency against ALK than crizotinib (Li et al., 2011) and activity in both crizotinib-sensitive and crizotinib-resistant tumors (Li et al., 2011; Marsilje et al., 2013). These encouraging results provided solid evidence to initiate a phase I study in the Western population, followed by an evaluation in Japanese patients.

2.2.6.1 Western Dose Escalation

The phase I study in Western patients was the first evaluation of ceritinib in humans with the primary objective: *To determine the MTD of LDK378 as a single agent when administered orally to adult patients with tumors characterized by genetic abnormalities in ALK* (Radona, Lin, Robson, Dai, Hailman, & Chica, 2010). All details of the study can be found in the published protocol (Radona, Lin, Robson, Dai, Hailman, & Chica, 2010), yet the most important points are described here.

The dose escalation used the Bayesian logistic regression with overdose control (see Section 2.2.3) using the criterion $P(\pi_d \geq 0.33) < 0.25$ to control overdosing. As an additional safety measure, a maximal increase of 100% from the current dose was allowed. Dose-limiting toxicities during the first 24 days (3 days PK run-in followed by a cycle of 21 days) were the primary endpoint to assess the tolerability. Selection of the next dose was determined during a dose-escalation teleconference between the sponsor and the investigators, based on the available toxicity information, including adverse events not qualifying as DLTs, PK, pharmacodynamic and efficacy information. Finally, for a dose to be declared as an MTD, at least six patients had to be evaluated at this dose, and it either had to have high probability (≥60%) for the DLT rate to be in the target interval (16%–33%), or otherwise, at least 21 patients had to have been evaluated on the study already.

Since no clinical data were available, preclinical toxicity studies were used to predict the expected safety in humans. On the basis of this prediction, the following provisional doses (in mg) were defined: 25, 50 (starting dose), 100, 200, 400, 600, 800, 1,000, and 1,250. Additionally, the protocol allowed to explore other, for example intermediate, doses depending on accumulating safety information (Radona, Lin, Robson, Dai, Hailman, & Chica, 2010). The wide dose range and an anticipated MTD of 1,000 mg as estimated from animal data revealed that patients in early cohorts could be exposed to subtherapeutic doses. Therefore, single-patient cohorts were allowed for low doses until some predefined safety measures were reached, upon which at least three patients were to be enrolled in each cohort.

The prior distribution for the logistic model parameters (based on preclinical data) was as follows:

$$\begin{pmatrix} \log(\alpha_W) \\ \log(\beta_W) \end{pmatrix} \sim BVN\left(\begin{pmatrix} -2.43 \\ 0.21 \end{pmatrix}, \begin{pmatrix} 3.30^2 & -0.63 \cdot 3.30 \cdot 0.76 \\ -0.63 \cdot 3.30 \cdot 0.76 & 0.76^2 \end{pmatrix}\right)$$

with reference dose $d^* = 350$. This prior covers a wide range of plausible values for the DLT rate and reflects the uncertainty due to the extrapolation from animals to humans. The prior mean (95% interval) and interval probabilities for the provisional doses are shown in Figure 2.1. The wide 95% intervals translate into a high probability of overdose (>25%) for doses above 200 mg. Therefore, doses up to and including 200 mg were allowed to start with according to the escalation with overdose control (EWOC) principle. On the basis of additional information from the preclinical experiments, the team decided to use 50 mg as the starting dose.

As mentioned in Section 2.2.2, a thorough investigation of the model using operating characteristics and data scenarios needs to be done. This information can be found in the study protocol (Radona, Lin, Robson, Dai, Hailman, & Chica, 2010) and is not shown here.

We will now discuss three actual dose-escalation decisions that reflect typical cases for phase I studies. The data for the three decisions are given in Table 2.2.

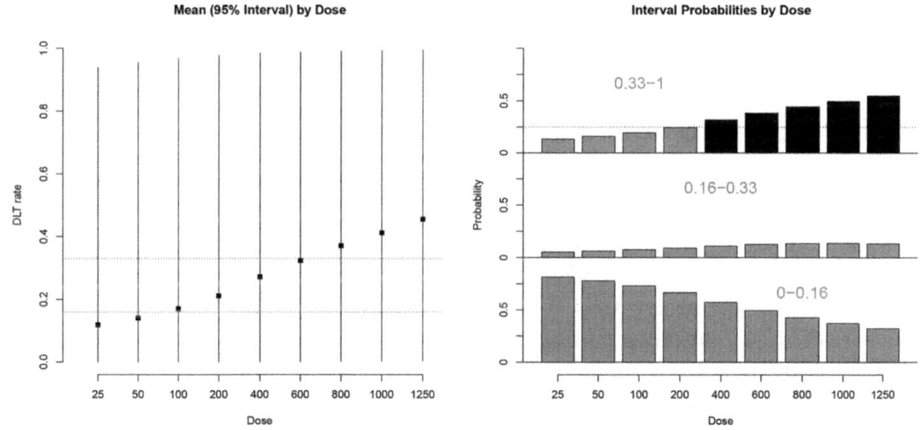

FIGURE 2.1
Prior distribution of DLT rate based on preclinical data.

TABLE 2.2

DLT Data at Different Decision Points in the Study

Decision	50	100	200	300	400	500	600	700	750
1	0/2	–	–	–	–	–	–	–	–
2	0/2	0/1	0/3	0/3	2/14	–	–	–	–
3	0/2	0/1	0/3	0/3	2/14	0/8	2/10	0/5	2/8

The first decision of interest is after the first cohort of patients at the lowest dose (50 mg) was enrolled. As allowed by the protocol, only two patients were enrolled at this dose, and none of them experienced a DLT. The dose-toxicity relationship is updated accordingly—the mean DLT rates are decreased compared to the prior, and the uncertainty (95% intervals) is reduced. As can be seen from Figure 2.2a, doses up to 500 mg were now eligible. However, due to the 100% escalation limit, the next dose chosen by the team was 100 mg.

The next decision was considered when the 400 mg dose had been studied in 14 patients, with 2 patients experiencing a DLT at 400 mg, but no DLTs occurred at lower doses. As expected, the 95% intervals became substantially narrower, and the means were updated reflecting the observed toxicity rate (Figure 2.2b). Doses up to 700 mg were eligible, which is sensible given that the observed DLT rate at 400 mg was only 21%, clearly below 33%. Interestingly, the team took a cautious approach at this point and decided to escalate only to 500 mg. It is likely that this was at least partially driven by safety considerations, including that 2 DLTs were observed at 400 mg.

Finally, we consider the decision at the end of the dose-escalation. In total, 59 patients were treated during the escalation, and 54 of them contributed to the dose-determining set. Overall, 6 DLTs occurred, all at or above 400 mg. At 750 mg, the highest DLT rate was observed (25%), yet due to the large number of patients, the uncertainty around the true DLT rates was low (Figure 2.2c), and all doses fulfilled the overdose control criterion. Even though further escalation had been possible, the team declared 750 mg as the MTD, based on additional safety information (Shaw et al., 2014).

2.2.6.2 Japanese Dose Escalation

Typically, a phase I study conducted in the Western population alone is considered insufficient by the Japanese Pharmaceuticals and Medical Devices Agency (PMDA) in order to initiate the clinical development in Japan. To assess the safety and tolerability of ceritinib in the Japanese population, a separate phase I study was therefore initiated (Nishio et al., 2015). In this situation, it is valuable to borrow information from the (likely on-going) Western study, which can be achieved using a MAC model. For example, we will discuss how such an analysis would look like when declaring the MTD for the Japanese study.

As discussed in Section 2.2.4, when using a MAC model (or any other approach to borrow information), it is important to assess the similarity between the trials. The more similar the studies are, the more homogeneous dose-toxicity profiles they should have, and the more willing we are to borrow information. Importantly, deciding about the similarity of the studies requires substantial input from clinicians. They know which patient factors potentially influence the dose-toxicity relationship and to what degree potentially different study populations can be assumed similar or not. For the case here, given the similarity of the two studies, it is reasonable

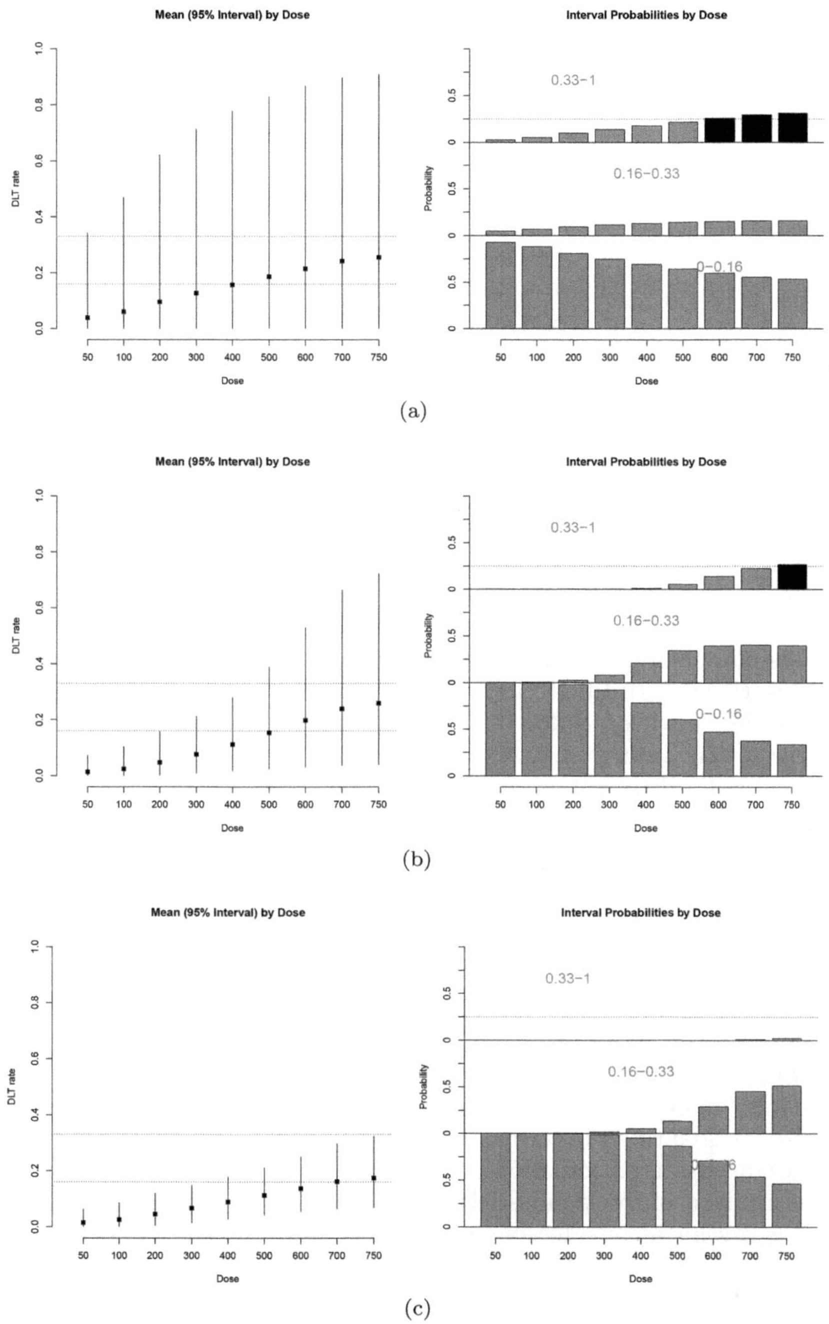

FIGURE 2.2
Analysis of Western study at three decision points. (a) Inference after first cohort. (b) Inference after doses up to 400 mg were studied. (c) Inference at the end of dose-escalation.

to assume moderate between-trial heterogeneity (median), but allowing for small to substantial values (95% interval). The other parameters are given weakly informative prior distributions (see Section 2.2.4), resulting in the following priors:

$$\tau_1 \sim LN\left(\log(0.25),(\log(2)/1.96)^2\right)$$

$$\tau_2 \sim LN\left(\log(0.125),(\log(2)/1.96)^2\right)$$

$$\mu_1 \sim N\left(\text{logit}(1/3),2^2\right)$$

$$\mu_2 \sim N\left(0,1^2\right)$$

$$\rho \sim U(-1,1)$$

In the Japanese study, the following doses (in mg) were explored: 300, 450, 600, and 700. The corresponding data are provided in Table 2.3. The dose-DLT profile in the Japanese patients seemed to be similar to that of the Western population, for which the data can be found in Table 2.2 (decision 3).

Figure 2.3a shows the results of the MAC analysis of the Japanese data. There is convincing evidence that all doses tested in Japanese patients are tolerable (EWOC fulfilled), and further escalation beyond 750 mg would be possible. However, as for the Western study, it does not imply that further escalation is necessary. Actually, in the Japanese phase I study (which used a slightly different approach to leverage the Western data), the team declared 750 mg as the MTD (Nishio et al., 2015), despite higher doses being eligible too.

For this case study, it is interesting to compare the MAC analysis to an analysis of the Japanese data alone using a weakly informative prior. The results of the latter are presented in Figure 2.3b. This analysis also reveals that all doses studied are tolerable, and the dose-toxicity profile (posterior means) looks similar to the one obtained from the MAC analysis. However, in comparison to the MAC analysis, the 95% credible intervals are wider, reflecting that no information from the Western study is used.

The information gain when borrowing information from the Western data can also be quantified in terms of *ESS*, for example, considering the 750 mg dose. Using the approximation described in Section 2.2.5, we find $ESS = 14$ for the analysis of the Japanese data alone and $ESS = 30$ for the MAC analysis. This reveals a considerable information gain to some extent due to the

TABLE 2.3

Japanese Study: DLT Data at Time of MTD Declaration

	300	450	600	750
DLT/N	0/3	0/6	1/4	1/7

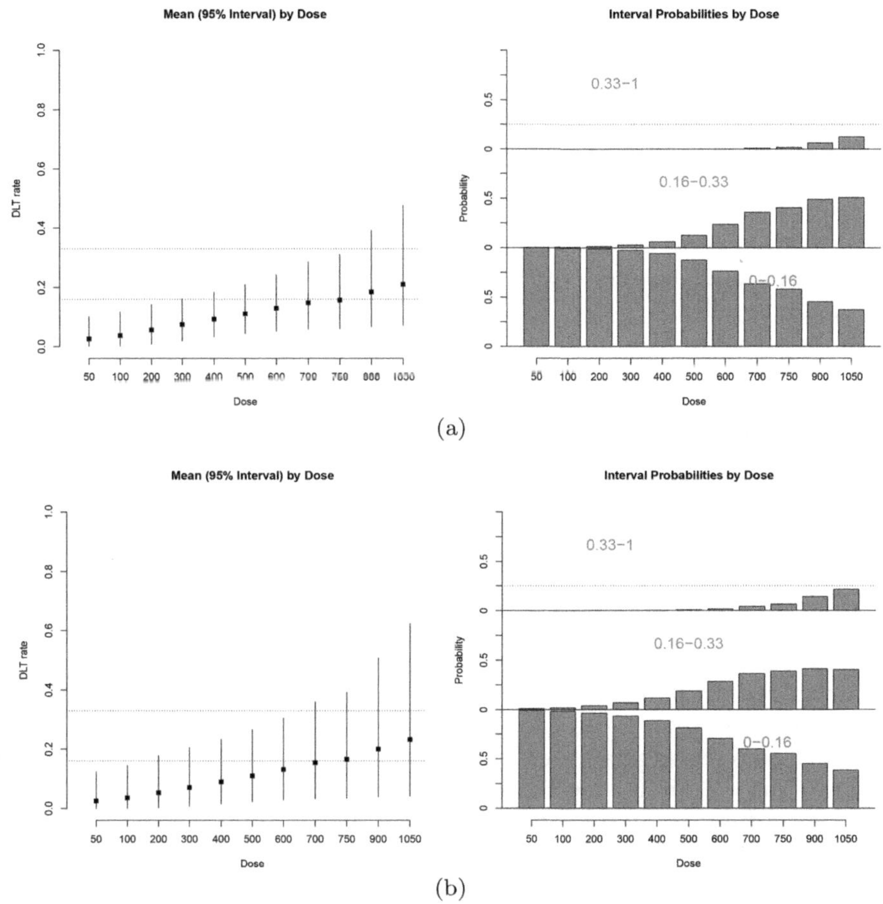

FIGURE 2.3
Analysis of Japanese study with and without Western data. (a) Analysis with Western data (MAC model). (b) Analysis without Western data

homogeneity of the study results. In case of more heterogeneous results, the information gain would be less due to the increased between-trial heterogeneity. This case could also be prospectively addressed using more robust models, as will be discussed in the next section.

Even when using a MAC model, we are interested in a summary of the prior DLT rate for the Japanese population, that is, before any Japanese data are available. We obtain this summary from the prior predictive distribution for the Japanese population given the Western data. Technically, there are different ways to sample from this distribution. We could either specify it explicitly in the model, or alternatively, we could use data from a Japanese cohort with arbitrary sample size but missing DLT data in the analysis. The latter may be a quicker (and simpler) approach, which is often applied in practice.

The Bayesian model-based approach described here has been implemented in more than 100 studies to date (Neuenschwander, Matano, Tang, Roychoudhury, Wandel, & Bailey, 2014). While this illustrates its broad applicability, it also reminds us that many phase I studies will not end with the dose escalation. Even when an MTD is defined, a lot of uncertainty remains about many aspects of the drug, including its general tolerability and potential efficacy. Therefore, it is quite popular nowadays to enroll additional patients during an expansion phase. In the next chapter, we will discuss the expansion phase more extensively and provide some approaches for its design and analysis.

2.3 Dose Expansion in Phase I Studies

As described in the introduction, the main objective of phase I studies in oncology is to evaluate the safety and tolerability of a new drug in a previously untested patient population. Historically, for cytotoxic agents, most responses were seen at doses close to the MTD. For example, von Hoff and Turner (Von Hoff & Turner, 1991) found that the majority of responses occurred within 80%–120% of the RP2D. Therefore, the MTD was often a promising dose from an efficacy perspective.

However, with targeted therapies, this paradigm has been questioned for several reasons. First, even though limited research on the topic has been conducted, there is evidence that responses may occur already at low doses (Jain et al., 2010). This, in turn, led to an increased awareness that an optimal dose, that is, a dose with good efficacy and low toxicity, rather than a maximal dose should be found (Roberts et al., 2004). Second, it is important to identify the right population using molecular data (Wong, Capasso, & Eckhardt, 2016), since targeted therapies have a much higher chance to work in these biologically selected groups. And third, especially for monoclonal antibodies and immune therapies, efficacy plays an important role in early clinical development (Postel-Vinay, Aspeslagh, Lanoy, Robert, Soria, & Marabelle, 2016).

The previous points illustrate why in recent years, an increasing number of phase I studies included one or multiple expansion cohorts to further study the selected dose (and regimen). For example, in a review of more than 600 phase I trials, Manji et al (Manji et al., 2013) found that about a quarter of the studies included an expansion cohort. Importantly, more recent trials used them more frequently. The objectives for the expansion cohorts included safety, efficacy, PK and pharmacodynamic evaluations, and patient enrichment. The latter specifically refers to the identification of patient populations for which a treatment benefit seems more likely than for an unselected population.

As one may imagine, in practice there is great heterogeneity in the actual conduct and implementation of dose-expansion cohorts. For example, in the studies investigated by Manji et al. (Manji et al., 2013), the median sample size was 17, with a range from 2 to 271 patients; other groups found similar results (Iasonos & O'Quigley, 2013; Dahlberg, Shapiro, Clark, & Johnson, 2014; Boonstra et al., 2015). Certainly, extreme cases with few hundred patients enrolled are uncommon and often driven by outstanding clinical efficacy, which may justify the collapse of a full clinical program into a single trial (Prowell, Theoret, & Pazdur, 2016).

Here, however, we will concentrate on the more common expansion phases, which include typically around 15–30 patients. The main goal of the section is twofold. In the first part, we aim to provide some practical advice for expansion phases that are mainly conducted for signal seeking. These are usually the smaller, more exploratory studies for drugs where much is still unknown, and clinical evidence needs to be generated in order to better understand and define the potential further development. In the second part, we discuss more rigorous designs for the expansion phase, including an indirect comparison in order to benchmark against competitor treatments. The latter may be particularly important since it illustrates how informed decision making can be supported already at a very early, yet critical stage in the drug development process.

2.3.1 Dose Expansion for Signal Seeking

We consider an example by Infante and colleagues (Infante et al., 2012) who published a phase I dose-escalation study with an expansion part in three different indications. The rationale for the expansion was multifold, including safety, efficacy, and PK objectives. This is typical for early phase studies where multiple aspects of the drug are of interest. In this situation, the expansion phase mainly serves the purpose of estimating a potential effect and quantifying the uncertainty associated with it. Still, however, it is important to provide some characteristics of the design in order to justify the sample size. This information is not only relevant for the sponsor, but also for review boards (e.g., ethics committees or regulatory agencies) that must decide whether the potential benefits outweigh the potential risks for patients.

Assessing a potential risk for patients can be particularly important since some endpoints may require that patients undergo additional, special procedures. For example, biopsies may be taken to assess biomarkers or scans may be performed for imaging purposes. The sample size for these procedures should then be justified on its own. This approach was followed by Infante and colleagues—a sample size justification for the safety objective and another one for the imaging objective was provided. We will consider these in more detail in the next sections.

2.3.1.1 Safety Endpoints

Infante et al. (Infante et al., 2012) provided the following sample size justification. *A cohort of 12 patients in the expansion tumor types provided a 72% likelihood of observing (at least once) a toxicity that has a true occurrence rate of at least 10%.* This statement reveals that the chosen sample size is sufficient to investigate the safety of the particular dose (and regimen) and allows some meaningful conclusions at the end of the study. Of course, the likelihood of 72% may look somewhat arbitrary. Therefore, in the study protocol, it may be worthwhile to show the same calculation for additional sample sizes and other true occurrence rates. Table 2.4 is an example of how this information could be presented. For a range of true occurrence rates and a number of sample sizes, the likelihood of observing at least one event is shown. The likelihood for the chosen sample size and true occurrence rate is highlighted in bold.

The information in the table provides a comprehensive picture of the interesting cases and as such, it can also be used during the design phase of the study. For example, when discussing the sample size with the clinical study team, it may be insightful to consider different options rather than just one specific case. For the study by Infante et al., we can imagine that a sample size of 15 could have been another obvious choice, with close to 80% likelihood of observing at least one event for a true rate of 0.10, and around 90% likelihood for a true rate of 0.15. Such considerations can help to reassure the team that the originally planned sample size has acceptable statistical properties, or, if that is not the case, to refine it accordingly.

2.3.1.2 Efficacy and Biomarker Endpoints

Infante and colleagues required a special imaging procedure (FDG-PET) for patients and they provided a rationale that the generated evidence is sufficient for the desired purpose. Importantly, for such endpoints (or similar ones, e.g., biomarker endpoints), we are typically more interested in estimating an effect rather than testing a formal hypothesis. The sample size justification should reflect that accordingly; for example, by considering the 95% confidence interval assuming a specific observed effect (point estimate). Infante et al. (2012) provided the following sample size justification for a

TABLE 2.4

Probability of Observing At Least One Adverse Event (AE) Depending on True AE Rate and Sample Size

AE rate	10	12	15	20
0.05	0.40	0.46	0.54	0.64
0.10	0.65	**0.72**	0.79	0.88
0.15	0.80	0.86	0.91	0.96
0.20	0.89	0.93	0.96	0.99

response rate based on FDG-PET imaging—*For FDG-PET, the observation of five or more metabolic responders in 20 patients would provide at least 95% confidence that the true metabolic response rate is more than 10%.* Again, we think it would be helpful to consider different scenarios and provide them in a table in the protocol, similar to what we propose for the safety endpoints (see Section 2.3.1.1). Furthermore, we generally prefer a two-sided rather than a one-sided confidence intervals. Accordingly, in Table 2.5, the point estimates and exact 95% confidence intervals are shown for different sample sizes and different observed response rates. In bold, the values corresponding to the sample size chosen by Infante et al. are highlighted. Again, as for the safety endpoint, this information may help to undermine the choice of the sample size while transparently showing other potential options.

2.3.2 Dose Expansion with a Formal Success Criterion for Efficacy

In some situations, the signal-seeking approach may be insufficient or inappropriate, for example, if the new drug under consideration is not first in class. In this case, we may have external evidence that a certain level of efficacy; that is, a clinically relevant effect should be reached in order to pursue further drug development. At the same time, if promising evidence is generated during the expansion phase, this may lead to an accelerated development and the immediate initiation of a phase III study. Due to their broad implications, such decisions should rely on a formal, predefined study success criterion for the expansion phase. Equally, however, the success criterion should reflect the early stage of development and thus be less rigorous than what we would use; for example, in a phase III study. Here, we will discuss two different designs that address these aspects.

2.3.2.1 Double Criterion Design

This design relies on a study success criterion that incorporates two different perspectives. The first is the clinical perspective—we claim success only if a

TABLE 2.5

Point Estimate and Exact 95% Confidence Interval for Different Observed Response Rates and Sample Sizes

Sample Size		
15	**20**	**25**
3 (20.0)	4 (20.0)	5 (20.0)
(4.3; 48.1)	(5.7; 43.7)	(6.8; 40.7)
4 (26.7)	**5 (25.0)**	6 (24.0)
(7.8; 55.1)	**(8.7; 49.1)**	(9.4; 45.1)
5 (33.3)	6 (30.0)	7 (28.0)
(11.8; 61.6)	(11.9; 54.3)	(12.1; 49.4)

minimally clinically relevant effect is obtained. The second is the statistical perspective—we control the risk of wrongly claiming success if, in reality, the treatment is ineffective. These perspectives are equally important, and the success criterion should, therefore, give equal weight to both of them.

Before formally defining the success criterion, it is important to understand the meaning of the minimally clinically relevant effect. The minimally clinically relevant effect is the threshold that separates a potentially interesting drug from a drug for which further development should not be considered. Only if we observe at least this effect, we are willing to initiate further development. Other authors refer to it as the *target difference* (Fisch, Jones, Jones, Kerman, Rosenkranz, & Schmidli, 2015), the *minimum clinically important difference* (Chuang-Stein, Kirby, Hirsch, & Atkinson, 2011), or the *critical threshold* (Neuenschwander, Rouyrre, Hollaender, Zuber, & Branson, 2011). Importantly, choosing the minimally clinically relevant effect requires a thorough understanding and review of the literature. We cannot emphasize enough the importance of this task, which is too often given insufficient consideration in practice.

For the formal definition of study success, we use a Bayesian double criterion as follows:

- Posterior median at least minimally clinically relevant (clinical perspective)
- Sufficiently large posterior probability to be better than a null effect (statistical perspective)

For the second criterion, we may reflect the early stage of development using a less stringent threshold than what we would use in a confirmatory-like study.

As an example, we consider an expansion phase with an objective response rate (ORR) as the primary endpoint. The available evidence is assumed to suggest an ORR of 25% being the minimal effect for considering further development. Moreover, we want to exclude that the true ORR is less than 15%, which would mean that the treatment is no better than the standard of care. We use p_T to denote the parameter of interest and define the double criterion as follows:

- Posterior median: $P(p_T \geq 0.25) \geq 0.5$
- Posterior probability: $P(p_T \geq 0.15) \geq 0.95$

The statistical model is beta-binomial with a weakly informative prior distribution $\theta \sim Beta(1/3, 1)$. This distribution has a mean of 0.25 and a wide 95% interval (0.00, 0.93) reflecting our uncertainty about p_T.

While we have now defined the statistical model and the success criterion, we still need to select an appropriate sample size. As for any early phase clinical trial, the choice of the sample size is not only based on statistical considerations but also influenced by other factors such as feasibility, competitive landscape, and financial aspects. However, the operating characteristics, that is, power and type I error, remain a key factor for determining the sample size.

By design, the type I error will be around 5%, regardless of the sample size. On the other hand, for the power calculation, the sample size is of course critical. We use $p_T = 0.35$ as an alternative effect for the power calculation. The corresponding power curve is shown in Figure 2.4. Due to the discrete sampling space, we obtain a sawtooth curve, which indicates a sample size $n = 31$ to achieve at least 80% power. This power curve helps in the selection of the sample size during the design phase and may also be presented in the appropriate section of the study protocol.

2.3.2.2 Single-Arm Design with Indirect Comparison to Comparator

Even when conducting a single-arm study, we inherently try to answer the following question: How would the new treatment compare to the current (or a future) standard of care, had the latter been included in the study? Often, we provide a simplified answer to this question, comparing the treatment effect against a fixed historical value. However, such an approach overlooks

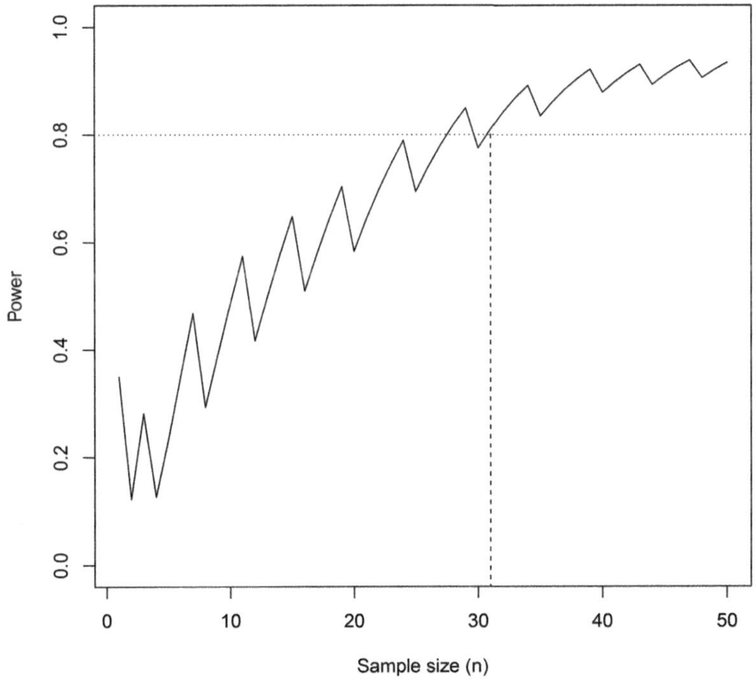

FIGURE 2.4
Power curve for double criterion design assuming $p_T = 0.35$.

two important uncertainties. The first is the uncertainty in the standard-of-care treatment effect (parameter uncertainty), which is completely ignored when only using a fixed value. The second is the uncertainty due to potential differences between studies, that is, the between-trial heterogeneity. When aiming to (best) compare the new treatment with the standard of care, we need to account for these uncertainties.

An approach that accounts for both uncertainty in parameter estimation and between-trial heterogeneity is the MAC approach (see Section 2.2.4). In order to illustrate it, we consider again an example using ORR as the endpoint of interest. As before, we will work in the Bayesian framework. Despite offering a natural way for making predictions, the Bayesian approach also helps in overcoming particular challenges with meta-analyses when the number of studies is small (Friede, Röver, Wandel, & Neuenschwander, 2016a,b). The latter may often be encountered in practice since the number of available studies on the standard of care can be quite limited.

Considering notation, for the treatment group, we denote the number of responses by $r_{*,T}$, the number of patients by $n_{*,T}$, and the true ORR by $p_{*,T}$, where the index * refers to the current study. For the control (i.e., the standard of care) group, we denote the number of responses in the i-th historical study by $r_{i,C}$, the number of patients by $n_{i,C}$, and the true ORR by $p_{i,C}$. Accordingly, $p_{*,C}$ denotes the (predicted) ORR for the control in the new study. The study success criterion uses now the quantities $p_{*,T}$ and $p_{*,C}$ as follows:

$$\text{Study success} = P\left(p_{\star,T} > p_{C,\star} \mid \text{Data}\right) \geq 0.80,$$

which means we require at least 80% posterior probability that the treatment is better than the (predicted) standard of care. The statistical model is given by:

$$r_{\star,T} \sim Bin\left(n_{\star,T}, p_{\star,T}\right)$$

$$r_{i,C} \sim Bin\left(n_{i,C}, p_{i,C}\right)$$

$$\text{logit}\left(p_{i,C}\right) \sim N\left(\mu, \tau^2\right)$$

$$\text{logit}\left(p_{\star,C}\right) \sim N\left(\mu, \tau^2\right)$$

with prior distributions

$$p_{\star,T} \sim Beta(2/3, 1)$$

$$\mu \sim N\left(0, 2^2\right) \quad .$$

$$\tau \sim \text{HN}(0.5)$$

Here, *HN*(0.5) denotes the half-Normal distribution with scale 0.5, that is, if $x \sim N\left(0, 0.5^2\right)$, then $\tau = |x| \sim \mathrm{HN}(0.5)$. The prior distribution for μ is weakly informative (see Section 2.2.4), and the prior distribution for τ has a median 0.34% and 95% interval (0.015, 0.12). On the logit scale, these values reflect moderate between-trial heterogeneity (median), and the 95% interval allows for small to large values; for more details, see (Neuenschwander, Matano, Tang, Roychoudhury, Wandel, & Bailey, 2014; Friede, Röver, Wandel, & Neuenschwander, 2016a,b). Finally, the Beta prior distribution for $p_{*,T}$ is weakly informative, with mean 40% and 95% interval (0.00, 0.96).

For the standard of care, data from two historical studies were available, shown in Table 2.6. In the same table, we also show the predicted ORR for the standard of care in the new study.

For this study, a maximal sample size of $n = 40$ for the expansion phase was deemed feasible by the clinical team. The minimal number of responders for study success, that is, to obtain $P\left(p_{\star,T} > p_{\star,C} \,|\, \mathrm{Data}\right) \geq 0.80$, is then $r_{\star,T} = 18$. This number can be found by evaluating the posterior probability for a number of consecutive values of $r_{*,T}$, until for the first time the success criterion is fulfilled.

Similar to the example in Section 2.3.2.1, we find a power curve that is informative to facilitate design discussions and would recommend to include it in the study protocol. However, while we plotted the power as a function of the sample size in the example of Section 2.3.2.1, we now plot it as a function of $p_{*,T}$ for a given sample size of $n = 40$. Figure 2.5 reveals that the power is close to 80% (or above) when assuming $p_{\star,T} = 50\%$ or above. On the other hand, for $p_{\star,T} = 30\%$ or below, the false-positive rate is at most 3.2%. These numbers provide reassurance that the sample size is adequately chosen considering realistic assumptions on the true (but unknown) response rate $p_{*,T}$.

2.3.3 Advanced Designs: Fully Hierarchical Models

The designs outlined previously may not always reflect the study setup appropriately. For example, in the expansion phase, multiple strata defined by tumor types may be enrolled in parallel. Or, enrollment in multiple strata based on biomarker expression may happen. In these situations (which are

TABLE 2.6

ORR Data from Historical Studies of Standard of Care and Prediction for New Study

Study	*r*/*n*	ORR (95% Interval) [Percentage]
1	19/52	36.5 (23.6–51.0)[a]
2	37/126	29.4 (21.6–38.1)[a]
* (New Study)	N/A	32.1 (14.4–59.6)[b]

[a] Frequentist point estimate and exact interval.
[b] Bayesian prediction: median and 95% interval.

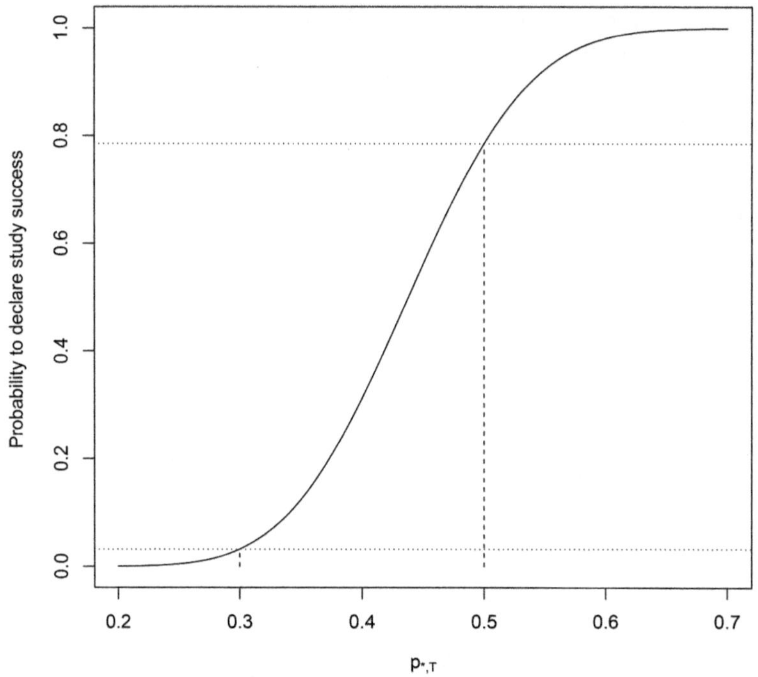

FIGURE 2.5
Study success probability for indirect comparison design ($n = 40$).

conceptually similar to BASKET trials (Redig & Jänne, 2015)), we may find that neither a pooled nor a stratified analysis adequately captures the underlying design. Rather, we would prefer a statistical model that allows the borrowing of information between strata while accounting for between-strata heterogeneity. Such a model will result in more precise strata-specific estimates as compared to those from a stratified analysis, without the strong assumptions underlying a pooled analysis. Bayesian hierarchical models have proven particularly useful in this context.

For example, Chugh et al. (2009) and similarly Schuetze et al. (2016) investigated multiple subtypes of sarcoma using a Bayesian hierarchical model developed by Thall et al. (Thall, Wathen, Bekele, Champlin, Baker, & Benjamin, 2013). A Bayesian hierarchical model (Zhou, Liu, & Kim, 2008) was also used in the Biomarker-integrated Approaches of Targeted Therapy for Lung Cancer Elimination program of personalized medicine (Kim et al., 2011) and in the Signature trial (Warsi et al., 2015). Even though the latter two examples had very large sample sizes, the underlying statistical principle could also be applied to an expansion phase. What all these examples have in common is that they rely on models that assume the strata-specific parameters θ_j to be exchangeable. Typically, this is achieved using a suitable transformation g, such that normality for $g(\theta_j)$ is plausible, resulting in hierarchical models of the following form:

$$g(\theta_j) \sim N(\mu, \tau^2),$$

with prior distributions for μ and τ, respectively.

Often, such hierarchical models may be adequate, especially when no dramatic differences between strata are expected. However, the advantage that these models offer can turn into a disadvantage when the exchangeability assumption is violated, typically when one stratum is very different from the others. This observation was made, for example, by Berry, Broglio, Groshen, and Berry (2013), and one way to address the problem is given in Leon-Novelo, Bekele, Müller, Quintana, and Wathen (2012). Another solution was proposed by Neuenschwander, Wandel, Ryochoudhury, & Bailey (2016), which can be interpreted as a robust exchangeability model. In this model, each stratum-specific parameter is assumed to belong to the exchangeable distribution only with probability p_j, and to follow a stand-alone distribution with the remaining probability $1 - p_j$. The above model thus translates into

$$\begin{aligned} g(\theta_j) &\sim N(\mu, \tau^2) \quad \text{with probability } p_j \\ g(\theta_j) &\sim N(m_j, s_j^2) \quad \text{with probability } 1 - p_j \end{aligned}$$

where m_j, s_j are strata-specific. An application of that model is also given in (Neuenschwander, Wandel, Ryochoudhury, & Bailey, 2016).

Finally, the effort required to design studies that use hierarchical models should not be underestimated. No standard software may be available for the analysis, and clinical trial simulation can become quite time-consuming. Furthermore, the implication of design changes, such as adding or removing strata, is incomparably larger than for non-hierarchical designs. These aspects should be accounted for and should be brought to the clinical team's awareness before a decision is made whether to use a hierarchical model or not.

2.4 Conclusion

The design and conduct of phase I trials in oncology has changed dramatically during the past few years. In the early days of cancer research, when mainly chemotherapies were used, the primary goal was to reach a high dose while avoiding a toxic dose. Clinical efficacy, selection of a targeted population, understanding signaling pathways, and optimization of dosing was not a primary focus in these days. Nowadays, however, these topics are highly relevant already in early development, and while finding a clinically acceptable (i.e., tolerable) dose is still important, it is only one of several goals in a phase I trial. The increased use of expansion phases (Manji et al., 2013) in more recent years reflects the trend to obtain efficacy signals early on to gain a broader (and better) understanding of many clinically important aspects. It is, therefore, no surprise that phase I trials are becoming statistically and operationally more complex and challenging for clinical teams.

Despite the trend to broaden the scope of phase I trials, the dose escalation remains one of their key components. Using a good model for dose escalation is important, and different proposals have been made in the literature; for an overview, see (Ivy, Siu, Garrett-Mayer, & Rubinstein, 2010). However, it would have gone beyond the scope of this chapter to introduce and discuss them in detail. Rather, we decided to describe the approach that has been used successfully at Novartis Oncology for more than 10 years now, and which has been implemented in over 100 studies (Neuenschwander, Matano, Tang, Roychoudhury, Wandel, & Bailey, 2014). Still, most of the considerations here apply to any dose escalation regardless of the approach that is used. Importantly, further extensions to the model have been proposed, and the interested reader is referred to Neuenschwander, Roychoudhury, and Schmidli (2016) and Neuenschwander, Wandel, Ryochoudhury, and Bailey (2016) for multi-strata designs, and to Cotterill, Lorand, Wang, and Jaki (2015) for the potential inclusion of PK data. Finally, the combination of two or more drugs is extensively discussed in Neuenschwander, Matano, Tang, Roychoudhury, Wandel, & Bailey, 2014 and an actual published study can be found in Bedard et al., 2015. Especially for drug combinations, we recommend the aforementioned pre-reads and would like to bring to the readers' awareness that unexpected toxicities can become a limiting factor in this setting (see e.g., Ribas, Hodi, Callahan, Konto, & Wolchok, 2013), which needs to be acknowledged beforehand.

In the second part of the chapter, we focused on the expansion phase, which is becoming increasingly important in practice. To our surprise, while there is a vast literature on the dose-escalation phase available, we could only identify a few articles dedicated to the expansion phase. Partially, this may be explained by the simplicity of the designs (single-arm, binary endpoint) often used for this phase. However, in our experience, the expansion phase comes with its own specific challenges, due to its hermaphrodite nature—on one hand, it still serves the exploratory purpose of early drug development, yet on the other hand, it is the base for far-reaching decisions. In this situation, traditional approaches for single-arm designs may be inadequate, and alternatives are required. Therefore, we discussed four different approaches, two for signal seeking and two for early efficacy assessment. However, it is also clear that study success (or failure) is not the only base for a decision on the future development of a compound. Such a result will always be reflected in the light of other, study-external evidence, something which is important for studies in any phase of development, including pivotal studies (Pocock & Stone, 2016a,b). As statisticians, it is, therefore, our task to anticipate how we can best support these decisions with evidence-based statements from the current study, whether these are inferential or descriptive only.

Finally, the approaches that we discussed are only a selection amongst many options. Also, they could be modified or extended where required. For example, the indirect comparison design could be generalized to more than one treatment, following the ideas outlined in Schmidli, Wandel, and Neuenschwander (2013). On the other hand, the signal-seeking approach could be extended to consider more than one endpoint simultaneously. The material in this chapter hopefully provides a useful source for such extensions and serves as the first stop for statisticians working on phase I trials in oncology.

Acknowledgments

We would like to thank Beat Neuenschwander and Heinz Schmidli for the many fruitful discussions on statistical–technical subjects, and Stuart Bailey and Michael Branson for their ongoing support in implementing Bayesian methods in practice.

Appendix

We provide R-code to re-run the analyses of section 2.2.6.

Single-Agent Model for Western Dose Escalation

```
# ---------------------------------------------------
# model definition
# ---------------------------------------------------
model_single <- function(){

  # covariance, precision matrix
  cov[1,1] <- Prior[3]*Prior[3]
  cov[2,2] <- Prior[4]*Prior[4]
  cov[1,2] <- Prior[3]*Prior[4]*Prior[5]
  cov[2,1] <- cov[1,2]
  prec[1:2,1:2] <- inverse(cov[,])

  # prior distribution
  logAB[1:2] ~dmnorm(Prior[1:2],prec[1:2,1:2])

  # likelihood
  for (i in 1:Ncohorts){
```

```
    logit(P1[i]) <- logAB[1]+exp(logAB[2])*log(DosesAdm[i]/
    DoseRef) Ntox[i]~dbin(P1[i],Npat[i])

  }

  # for output
  # probabilities of toxicity: P
  # pCat is an indicator corresponding to toxicity categories
  # the respective means correspond to interval probabilities
  for(i in 1:Ndoses){

    logit(P[i]) <- logAB[1]+exp(logAB[2])*log(Doses[i]/DoseRef)
    for (j in 1:Nint){
      Pcat[i,j] <- step(P[i] - Pcutoffs[j])*step(Pcutoffs[j+1]
      - P[i])
    }
    # prediction
    NtoxPred[i]~dbin(P[i], NewCohortSize)

    # predictive probability of 0:NewCohortSize toxicities
    for (j in 0:NewCohortSize) {
      pred.Tox[i,j+1] <- equals(NtoxPred[i],j)
    }
  }
}

# ------------------------------------------------
# actual analysis
# ------------------------------------------------
library(R2WinBUGS)

 fixed <- list(
  Prior = c(-2.43, 0.21, 3.3, 0.76, -0.63),
  Nint = 3,
  Pcutoffs = c(0,0.16, 0.33,1)
)
 inits <- list(
  list( logAB = c(-2.0, -0.2) ), list( logAB = c(-2.0,  0.2)
),
  list( logAB = c( 0.0, -0.2) ), list( logAB = c( 0.0,  0.2) )
)

# ------------------------------------------------
# Prior - use a "trick" (prior predictive
# distribution for arbitrary dose, note that
# Ncohorts = 1 ensures the data for the second
# cohort are ignored)
# ------------------------------------------------
prior.data <- list(
  Ncohorts = 1,
```

```
  DosesAdm = c(50, 100),
  Ntox     = c(NA,   1),
  Npat     = c(3, 3),
  Ndoses   = 9,
  Doses = c(25, 50, 100, 200, 400, 600, 800, 1000, 1250),
  DoseRef = 350,
  NewCohortSize = 3
)
 prior.west <- bugs(
  data = c(fixed, prior.data),
  inits = inits,
  parameters.to.save = c("NtoxPred", "Pcat", "P"),
  model.file = model_single,
  n.iter = 25000,
  n.burnin = 5000,
  n.thin = 1,
  n.chains = 4,
  DIC = FALSE,
  summary.only = TRUE
)
# ---------------------------------------------------
# posterior summary
# ---------------------------------------------------
round(prior.west$stats, 3)
```

Meta-Analytic Combined Model for Western and Japanese Data

```
# ---------------------------------------------------
# model definition
# ---------------------------------------------------
model <- function(){

  # prior input: derive precision from standard deviation
  muA.prec <- pow(Prior.muA[2], -2)
  muB.prec <- pow(Prior.muB[2], -2)
  prec.tauA <- pow(Prior.tauA[2], -2)
  prec.tauB <- pow(Prior.tauB[2], -2)

  # priors for means of exchangeable distribution
  mu[1] ~dnorm(Prior.muA[1], muA.prec)
  mu[2] ~dnorm(Prior.muB[1], muB.prec)

  # priors for between-trial heterogeneity and correlation
  log.tau[1]~dnorm(Prior.tauA[1], prec.tauA)
  log.tau[2]~dnorm(Prior.tauB[1], prec.tauB)
  tau[1] <- exp(log.tau[1])
  tau[2] <- exp(log.tau[2])
  rho~dunif(Prior.rho[1],Prior.rho[2])

  # covariance, precision matrix
```

```
  cov[1,1]       <- pow(tau[1],2)
  cov[2,2]       <- pow(tau[2],2)
  cov[1,2]       <- tau[1]*tau[2]*rho
  cov[2,1]       <- cov[1,2]
  prec[1:2,1:2] <- inverse(cov[1:2,1:2])

  # vector of zeros
  zeros[1] <- 0
  zeros[2] <- 0

  # strata-specific parameters (meta-analytic, i.e.
hierarchical model)
  # j refers to stratum
  for (j in 1:Nstrata) {

    re[j,1:2]~dmnorm(zeros[1:2],prec[1:2,1:2])
    logAB[j,1] <- mu[1]+re[j,1]
    logAB[j,2] <- mu[2]+re[j,2]
  }

  # likelihood
  for (i in 1:Ncohorts){
    logit(P1[i]) <- logAB[Stratum[i],1] +
                    exp(logAB[Stratum[i],2])*log(DosesAdm[i]/
                    DoseRef)
    Ntox[i]~dbin(P1[i],Npat[i])
  }

  # for output
  # probabilities of toxicity: P
  # pCat is an indicator corresponding to toxicity categories
  # the respective means correspond to interval probabilities
  for (j in 1:Nstrata) {
    for (i in 1:Ndoses) {

      logit(P[j,i]) <- logAB[j,1]+exp(logAB[j,2])*log(Doses[i]/
      DoseRef)
      for (k in 1:Nint){
        Pcat[j,i,k] <- step(P[j,i] -
Pcutoffs[k])*step(Pcutoffs[k+1] - P[j,i])
      }

      # prediction
      NtoxPred[j,i]~dbin(P[j,i], NewCohortSize)

      # predictive probability of 0:NewCohortSize toxicities
      for (k in 0:NewCohortSize) {
        pred.Tox[j,i,k+1] <- equals(NtoxPred[j,i],k)
      }
    }
```

```
  }
}
# ---------------------------------------------------
# specification for Japanese MAC analysis
# ---------------------------------------------------
source("model_mac.R")
mac.fixed <- list(
  Prior.muA  = c(-0.693, 2),
  Prior.muB = c(0, 1),
  Prior.tauA = c(log(0.25), log(2)/1.96),
  Prior.tauB = c(log(0.125), log(2)/1.96),
  Prior.rho = c(-1,1),
  Nint = 3,
  Pcutoffs = c(0,0.16, 0.33, 1),
  Ndoses = 11,
  Doses = c(50, 100, 200, 300, 400, 500, 600, 700, 750, 900,
1050),
  DoseRef = 350
)

 mac.inits <- list(
  list( mu = c(-0.80, -0.2) ), list( mu = c(-0.80,  0.0) ),
  list( mu = c(-0.30,  0.5) ), list( mu = c(-2.50, -0.4) )
)

# ---------------------------------------------------
# MAC analysis at time of MTD declaration
# ---------------------------------------------------
mac.data <- list(
  Nstrata = 2,
  Ncohorts = 13,
  DosesAdm = c(50, 100, 200, 300, 400, 500, 600, 700, 750,
300, 450, 600, 750),
  Ntox =      c( 0,   0,   0,   0,   2,   2,   0,   0,   2,
0,   0,   1,   1),
  Npat =      c( 2,   1,   3,   3,  14,   8,  10,   5,   8,
3,   6,   4,   7),
  Stratum =  c( 1,   1,   1,   1,   1,   1,   1,   1,   1,
2,   2,   2,   2),
  NewCohortSize = 3
)

 mac.final <- bugs(
  data = c(mac.fixed, mac.data),
  inits = mac.inits,
  parameters.to.save = c("NtoxPred", "Pcat", "P"),
  model.file = model_mac,
  n.iter = 25000,
  n.burnin = 5000,
  n.thin = 1,
```

```
  n.chains = 4,
  DIC = FALSE,
  summary.only = TRUE
)

 # ---------------------------------------------------
# posterior summary; strata 2 = Japan
# ---------------------------------------------------
round(mac.final$stats, 3)
```

MAC Model for Binomial Data

```
# ---------------------------------------------------
# model definition
# ---------------------------------------------------
model_binom_MAC <- function(){

  # treatment: likelihood, prior
  rt~dbin(pt, nt)
  pt~dbeta(t.ab[1], t.ab[2])

  # standard of care: data from identified studies
  for(i in 1:ns){
    rc[i]~dbin(pc[i], nc[i])
    logit(pc[i]) <- theta[i]
    theta[i]~dnorm(mu, tau2.inv)
  }

  # standard of care: predicted effect for new study
  theta.pred~dnorm(mu, tau2.inv)
  logit(pc.pred) <- theta.pred

  # standard of care: priors for hierarchical model
  mu.prec <- pow(Prior.mu[2], -2)
  mu~dnorm(Prior.mu[1], mu.prec)

  tau2.inv <- pow(tau, -2)
  tau <- abs(tau.base)
  tau.base~dnorm(0, tau.scale2.inv)
  tau.scale2.inv <- pow(tau.scale, -2)

  # success is defined as: pt>pc.pred
  trt.suc <- step(pt - pc.pred)
 }

# ---------------------------------------------------
# specification for binomial MAC model
# ---------------------------------------------------

MACbinom.fixed <- list(
```

```
  t.ab = c(0.667, 1),
  Prior.mu = c(0, 2),
  tau.scale = 0.5
)

 MACbinom.inits <- list(
  list( mu =  0.5, tau.base = 0.1 ), list( mu = 0.5, tau.base
  = 0.1 ),
  list( mu = -0.5, tau.base = 0.2 ), list( mu = 0.5, tau.base
  = 0.2 )
)

# -----------------------------------------------------
# Analysis for data scenario: 18 responses out of
# 40 patients - just successful
# -----------------------------------------------------
MACbinom.data <- list(
  rt = 18,
  nt = 40,
  ns = 2,
  rc = c(19,  37),
  nc = c(52, 126)
)

 mac.binom.sc <- bugs(
  data = c(MACbinom.fixed, MACbinom.data),
  inits = MACbinom.inits,
  parameters.to.save = c("trt.suc", "pt", "pc.pred"),
  model.file = model_binom_MAC,
  n.iter = 25000,
  n.burnin = 5000,
  n.thin = 1,
  n.chains = 4,
  DIC = FALSE,
  summary.only = TRUE
)
 print(round(map.binom.sc$stats, 3))
```

References

Babb, J., Rogatko, A., & Zacks, S. (1998). Cancer phase I clinical trials: efficient dose escalation with overdose control. *Stat Med, 17* (10), 1103–20.

Bedard, P. L., Tabernero, J., Janku, F., Wainberg, Z. A., Paz-Ares, L., Vansteenkiste, J., ... Sessa, C. (2015). A phase Ib dose-escalation study of the oral Pan-PI3K inhibitor buparlisib (BKM120) in combi- nation with the oral MEK1/2 inhibitor trametinib (GSK1120212) in patients with selected advanced solid tumors. *Clin Cancer Res, 21* (4), 1103–20.

Berry, S., Broglio, K., Groshen, S., & Berry, D. (2013). Bayesian hierarchical modeling of patient subpopulations: efficient designs of Phase II oncology clinical trials. *Clin Trials, 10*(5), 720–34.

Boonstra, P., Shen, J., Taylor, J., Braun, T., Griffith, K., Daignault, S., ... Schipper, M. (2015). A statistical evaluation of dose expansion cohorts in phase I clinical trials. *J Natl Cancer Inst, 107*(3).

Chuang-Stein, C., Kirby, S., Hirsch, I., & Atkinson, G. (2011). The role of the minimum clinically important difference and its impact on designing a trial. *Pharm Stat, 10* (3), 250–6.

Chugh, R., Wathen, J., Maki, R., Benjamin, R., Patel, S., Meyers, P., ... Baker, L. (2009). Phase II multicenter trial of imatinib in 10 histologic subtypes of sarcoma using a Bayesian hierarchical statistical model. *J Clin Oncol, 27*(19), 3148–53.

Cotterill, A., Lorand, D., Wang, J., & Jaki, T. (2015). A practical design for a dual-agent dose-escalation trial that incorporates pharmacokinetic data. *Stat Med, 34*(13), 2138–64.

Dahlberg, S., Shapiro, G., Clark, J., & Johnson, B. (2014). Evaluation of statistical designs in phase I expansion cohorts: the Dana-Farber/Harvard Cancer Center experience. *J Natl Cancer Inst, 106*(7).

Eisenhauer, E. A., Twelves, C., & Buyse, M. (2006). *Phase I Cancer Trials – A Practical Approach*. Oxford University Press, Oxford, UK.

Fisch, R., Jones, I., Jones, J., Kerman, J., Rosenkranz, G., & Schmidli, H. (2015). Bayesian design of proof-of-concept trials. *Ther Innovation Regul Sci, 49*(1), 155–62.

Friede, T., R¨over, C., Wandel, S., & Neuenschwander, B. (2016a). Meta-analysis of few small studies in orphan diseases. Research Synthesis Methods. Retrieved from http://dx.doi.org/10.1002/jrsm.1217 (RSM-09–2015–0047.R1).

Friede, T., R¨over, C., Wandel, S., & Neuenschwander, B. (2016b). Meta-analysis of two studies in the presence of heterogeneity with applications in rare diseases. *Biom J, 59*(4), 658–71.

Iasonos, A., & O'Quigley, J. (2013). Design considerations for dose-expansion cohorts in phase I trials. *J Clin Oncol, 31* (33), 40144021.

Infante, J., Camidge, D., Mileshkin, L., Chen, E., Hicks, R., Rischin, D., ... Siu, L. (2012). Safety, pharmacokinetic, and pharmacodynamic phase I dose-escalation trial of PF-00562271, an inhibitor of focal adhesion kinase, in advanced solid tumors. *J Clin Oncol, 30*(13), 152733.

Ivy, S., Siu, L., Garrett-Mayer, E., & Rubinstein, L. (2010). Approaches to phase 1 clinical trial design focused on safety, efficiency, and selected patient populations: a report from the clinical trial design task force of the national cancer institute investigational drug steering committee. *Clin Cancer Res, 16*(6), 172636.

Jain, R., Lee, J., Hong, D., Markman, M., Gong, J., Naing, A., ... Kurzrock, R. (2010). Phase I oncology studies: evidence that in the era of targeted therapies patients on lower doses do not fare worse. *Clin Cancer Res, 16*(4), 1289–97.

Jaki, T., Clive, S., & Weir, C. (2013). Principles of dose-finding studies in cancer: a comparison of trial designs. *Cancer Chemother Pharmacol*, 71, 1107–14.

Kim, E., Herbst, R., Wistuba, I., Lee, J., Blumenschein, G., Tsao, A., ... Hong, W. (2011). The BATTLE trial: personalizing therapy for lung cancer. *Cancer Discov, 1*(1), 44–53.

Kwak, E., Bang, Y., Camidge, D., Shaw, A., Solomon, B., Maki, R., ... Iafrate, A. (2010). Anaplastic lymphoma kinase inhibition in non-small-cell lung cancer. *N Engl J Med, 363*(18), 1693–703.

Le Tourneau, C., Lee, J., & Siu, L. (2009). Dose escalation methods in phase I cancer clinical trials. *J Natl Cancer Inst, 101*(10), 708–20.

Le Tourneau, C., Razak, A., Gan, H., Pop, S., Di´eras, V., Tresca, P., & Paoletti, X. (2011). Heterogeneity in the definition of dose-limiting toxicity in phase I cancer clinical trials of molecularly targeted agents: a review of the literature. *Eur J Cancer, 47*(10), 1468–75.

Leon-Novelo, L., Bekele, N., Müller, P., Quintana, F., & Wathen, K. (2012). Borrowing Strength with Nonexchangeable Priors over Subpopulations. *Biometrics, 68*, 550–8.

Li, N., Michellys, P.-Y., Kim, S., Pferdekamper, A. C., Li, J., Kasibhatla, S., ... Harris, J. (2011). Abstract B232: Activity of a potent and selective phase I ALK inhibitor LDK378 in naive and crizotinib-resistant preclinical tumor models. *Mol Cancer Ther, 10* (1 suppl), B232.

Manji, A., Brana, I., Amir, E., Tomlinson, G., Tannock, I. F., Bedard, P. L., ... Razak, A. R. (2013). Evolution of clinical trial design in early drug development: systematic review of expansion cohort use in single-agent phase I cancer trials. *J Clin Oncol, 31*(33), 4260–7.

Marsilje, T. H., Pei, W., Chen, B., Lu, W., Uno, T., Jin, Y., ... Michellys, P. Y. (2013). Synthesis, structure-activity relationships, and in vivo efficacy of the novel potent and selective anaplastic lymphoma kinase (ALK) inhibitor 5-chloro-N2-(2-isopropoxy-5-methyl-4-(piperidin-4-yl)phenyl)-N4-(2-(isopropylsulfonyl) phenyl)pyrimidine-2,4-diamine (LDK378) currently in phase 1 and phase 2 clinical trials. *J Med Chem, 14*(56), 5675–90.

Morita, S., Thall, P., & Müller, P. (2008). Determining the effective sample size of a parametric prior. *Biometrics, 64*(2), 595–602.

Morita, S., Thall, P., & Müller, P. (2012). Prior effective sample size in conditionally independent hierarchical models. *Bayesian Anal, 7*(3), 591–614.

Neuenschwander, B., Branson, M., & Gsponer, T. (2008). Critical aspects of the Bayesian approach to phase I cancer trials. *Stat Med, 27*(13), 2420–39.

Neuenschwander, B., Capkun-Niggli, G., Branson, M., & Spiegelhalter, D. (2010). Summarizing historical information on controls in clinical trials. *Clin Trials, 7*(1), 5–18.

Neuenschwander, B., Matano, A., Tang, Z., Roychoudhury, S., Wandel, S., & Bailey, S. (2014). Statistical methods in drug combination studies. In W. Zhao & H. Yang (Eds.), chap. *A Bayesian Industry Approach to Phase I Combination Trials in Oncology*. Chapman and Hall/CRC.

Neuenschwander, B., Rouyrre, N., Hollaender, N., Zuber, E., & Branson, M. (2011). A proof of concept phase II non-inferiority criterion. *Stat Med, 30*(13), 1618–27.

Neuenschwander, B., Roychoudhury, S., & Schmidli, H. (2016). On the use of co-data in clinical trials. *Stat Biopharm Res, 8*(3), 345–54.

Neuenschwander, B., Wandel, S., Ryochoudhury, S., & Bailey, S. (2016). Ro-bust exchangeability designs for early phase clinical trials with multiple strata. *Pharm Stat, 15*(2), 123–34.

Nie, L., Rubin, E., Mehrotra, N., Pinheiro, J., Fernandes, L., Roy, A., ... de Alwis, D. (2016). Rendering the 3+3 design to rest: more efficient approaches to oncology dose-finding trials in the era of targeted therapy. *Clin Cancer Res, 22*(11), 2623–9.

Nishio, M., Murakami, H., Horiike, A., Takahashi, T., Hirai, F., Suenaga, N. T., S., ... (2015). Phase I study of ceritinib (LDK378) in Japanese Patients with advanced, anaplastic lymphoma kinase-rearranged non- small-cell lung cancer or other tumors. *J Thorac Oncol, 10*(7), 1058–66.

Pocock, S., & Stone, G. (2016a). The primary outcome fails – What next? *N Engl J Med, 375*(9), 861–70.
Pocock, S., & Stone, G. (2016b). The primary outcome is positive – Is that good enough? *N Engl J Med, 375*(10), 971–9.
Postel-Vinay, S., Aspeslagh, S., Lanoy, E., Robert, C., Soria, J. C., & Marabelle, A. (2016). Challenges of phase 1 clinical trials evaluating immune checkpoint-targeted antibodies. *Ann Oncol, 27*(2), 214–24.
Prowell, T., Theoret, M., & Pazdur, R. (2016). Seamless oncology-drug development. *N Engl J Med, 374*(21), 2001–3.
Radona, M., Lin, L., Robson, M., Dai, D., Hailman, E., & Chica, S. (2010). A phase I, multicenter, open-label dose escalation study of LDK378, administered orally in adult patients with tumors characterized by genetic abnormalities in anaplastic lymphoma kinase (ALK). Retrieved from http://www.nejm.org/doi/suppl/10.1056/NEJMoa1311107/suppl_file/nejmoa1311107_protocol.pdf
Redig, A., & J änne, P. (2015). Basket trials and the evolution of clinical trial design in an era of genomic medicine. *J Clin Oncol, 33*(9), 975–7.
Ribas, A., Hodi, F., Callahan, M., Konto, C., & Wolchok, J. (2013). Hepatotoxicity with combination of vemurafenib and ipilimumab. *N Engl J Med, 368*(14), 1365–6.
Riviere, M., Le Tourneau, C., Paoletti, X., Dubois, F., & Zohar, S. (2015). Designs of drug-combination phase I trials in oncology: a systematic review of the literature. *Ann Oncol, 26*(4), 669–74.
Roberts, T., Goulart, B., Squitieri, L., Stallings, S., Halpern, E., Chabner, B., ... Clark, J. (2004). Trends in the risks and benefits to patients with cancer participating in phase 1 clinical trials. *JAMA, 292*(17), 2130–40.
Schmidli, H., Gsteiger, S., Roychoudhury, S., O'Hagan, A., Spiegelhalter, D., & Neuenschwander, B. (2014). Robust meta-analytic-predictive priors in clinical trials with historical control information. *Biometrics, 70*(4), 1023–32.
Schmidli, H., Wandel, S., & Neuenschwander, B. (2013). The network meta-analytic-predictive approach to non-inferiority trials. *Stat Methods Med Res, 22*(2), 219–40.
Schuetze, S., Wathen, J., Lucas, D., Choy, E., Samuels, B., Staddon, A., ... Baker, L. (2016). SARC009: Phase 2 study of dasatinib in patients with previously treated, high-grade, advanced sarcoma. *Cancer, 122*(6), 868–74.
Shaw, A. T., Kim, D. W., Mehra, R., Tan, D. S., Felip, E., Chow, L. Q., ... Engelman, J. (2014). Ceritinib in ALK-rearranged non-small-cell lung cancer. *N Engl J Med, 370*(13), 1189–97.
Shaw, A. T., Kim, D. W., Nakagawa, K., Seto, T., Crinó, L., Ahn, M., ... J¨anne, P. (2013). Crizotinib versus chemotherapy in advanced ALK- positive lung cancer. *N Engl J Med, 368*(25), 2385–94.
Storer, B. (1989). Design and analysis of phase I clinical trials. *Biometrics, 45*(3), 925–37.
Thall, P., Wathen, J., Bekele, B., Champlin, R., Baker, L., & Benjamin, R. (2013). Hierarchical Bayesian approaches to phase II trials in diseases with multiple subtypes. *Stat Med, 22*(5), 763–80.
Von Hoff, D. D., & Turner, J. (1991). Response rates, duration of response, and dose response effects in phase I studies of antineoplastics. *Invest New Drugs, 9*(1), 115–22.
Wandel, S., Schmidli, H., & Neuenschwander, B. (2016). Cancer clinical trials: Current and controversial issues in design and analysis. In S. L. George, W. Wang, & H. Pang (Eds.), chap. *Use of Historical Data*. Chapman and Hall/CRC.

Warsi, G., Viele, K., Lebedinsky, C., Sudha, P., Slosberg, E., Kang, B., ... Berry, D. (2015). Bring the protocol to the patient. Retrieved 2017-01-02, from http://www.bayes-pharma.org/wp-content/uploads/2014/10/P2P-Signature-slides-for-Bayes-2015.pdf.

Wong, K., Capasso, A., & Eckhardt, S. (2016). The changing landscape of phase I trials in oncology. *Nat Rev Clin Oncol, 13*(2), 106–17.

Zhou, X., Liu, S., & Kim, E. (2008). Bayesian adaptive design for targeted therapy development in lung cancer – a step toward personalized medicine. *Clin Trials, 5*, 18–93.

3

Exposure–Response Analysis in Oncology Trials

Yi-Lin Chiu and Balakrishna S. Hosmane
AbbVie Inc.

CONTENTS

This chapter discusses and illustrates the following case studies from oncology:

3.1 Investigation of QT/QTc Prolongation
3.2 Bioequivalence (BE) Study in Cancer Patients Using Group Sequential Design

3.1 Investigation of QT/QTc Prolongation

3.1.1 Introduction

Maintaining proper cardiac function in patients undergoing cancer treatments is a concern in the development of any new drug. Cardiac safety has become a vital issue for cancer patients as the life expectancies are increased with emerging therapies. However, a thorough QT study design with placebo and active controls may not always be feasible; for instance, it is unethical to give placebo and/or active control (such as moxifloxacin) to cancer patients in the absence of a therapeutic benefit, while it is unsafe to administer a supra-therapeutic dose or even a therapeutic dose of a cytotoxic drug to healthy volunteers. To investigate the effect of an oncology compound on QT prolongation in patients, a high-precision QT study would still be advisable. Here, we show that with a carefully planned randomized crossover design in patients, the drug effect on QT prolongation can be estimated by the intersection–union test and exposure–response analysis.

3.1.2 Methodology

A phase 1, single-dose, open-label, randomized study in subjects with advanced solid tumors was conducted on 24 patients. This study was performed in accordance with the ethical standards laid down in the Declaration of Helsinki.[1] All patients gave their informed consent prior to participation in the study. Eligibility included age >18 years, ECOG performance status scores of 0–1, and adequate organ function. For the assessment of ECGs, patients were randomly assigned to two sequences of regimens of linifanib at the maximum tolerated dose (MTD), 0.25 mg/kg, without exceeding 17.5 mg, administered orally in a two-period (Day 1 and Day 7) crossover fashion. Subjects were administered a single morning dose under fasting or non-fasting conditions.

A single 12-lead resting ECG was obtained within the week before Day 1, or on Day 1, and on study completion or upon subject discontinuation. Triplicate ECGs were obtained serially on Day 1 at the anticipated time points for subsequent dosing, and before and after dosing on Day 1 and Day 7 (crossover Period 1 and Period 2, respectively). The time points for measurements were pre-dose and 0.5, 1, 2, 3, 4, 6, 8, 10, 12, and 24 h post-dose. Measurements were taken after the subject had been supine for 5 minutes. Pharmacokinetic plasma samples were also collected for 72h on Day 1 and Day 7.

QT, RR, PR and QRs intervals[2] were measured for each ECG using AbbVie's validated PC-based algorithm (ABBIOS), with standardized manual over-reading of all ECGs by trained technicians and T-U morphology assessment by cardiologists. QTc was determined using Fridericia's correction method[3] (QTcF):

$$QT_F = \frac{QT}{\sqrt[3]{RR}}$$

Values for the triplicate ECGs were averaged to obtain a single interval measurement for each time point.

3.1.2.1 Intersection–Union Test

A linear mixed effects model was used for the analysis of the Day 1 and Day 7 data to evaluate the effect of linifanib on cardiac repolarization. The analysis was performed for time-matched baseline-adjusted QTcF intervals (QTcF). For the assessment of the effect of linifanib, the primary endpoint was the largest time-matched difference for QTcF between drug regimens and baseline (ΔQTcF). An intersection–union test was performed at a significance level of 0.05 within the framework of the corresponding mixed effects model. Linifanib was considered to have a negative effect (not clinically significant effect) on cardiac repolarization if at all time points of the ECG measurements, the mean QTcF for linifanib did not exceed the baseline mean by 10ms or more with a statistical significance level of 0.05. Therefore, the maximum 95% upper confidence bound for the baseline-adjusted QTcF (ΔQTcF) must be less than 10ms in order to demonstrate a negative QTc effect. The intersection–union test required high operational and statistical precision of the data to meet the criteria for negative QT effect since the confidence intervals (CIs) would be narrower with tighter variability.

3.1.2.2 Exposure–Response Analysis

The relationship between baseline-adjusted QTcF and plasma drug concentration was also explored using an exposure–response analysis.

The model for the response variable QTcF is:

$$\text{QTcF} = \text{Intercept} + \beta_1\text{BaselineQTcF} + \beta_2\text{Concentration} + \text{SEQUENCE} + \text{DAY} + \text{HOUR} + \eta + \varepsilon.$$

The model has terms for baseline measurement (BaselineQTcF), sequence (SEQUENCE), day of measurement (DAY), and time of measurement (HOUR). The effects SEQUENCE, DAY, and HOUR are defined by classification rather than a quantitative measurement. A covariance structure for the data to account for correlation among observations within a subject is specified by modeling the subject-specific random variable η and the residual error ε. Within the framework of this model, the 95% upper confidence bound for the effect of the mean C_{max} of the linifanib dose on the QTcF was provided. If the bound is less than 10 ms, the regimen does not have a clinically relevant effect on cardiac repolarization.

3.1.3 Results and Conclusion

Twenty-four subjects were included in the QTcF analysis. No subject had QTcF values greater than 500 ms and no subject had a change greater than 60 ms from baseline. One subject had an asymptomatic QTcF change of greater than 30 ms from baseline.

Among the study population, baseline QTcF values ranged from 360.9 ms to 468.6 ms. After patients received linifanib, the ΔQTcF for the fasting regimen ranged from −4.14 ms to 0.64 ms, whereas the non-fasting regimen ranged from −6.03 ms to −1.57 ms (Table 3.1). The maximum 95% upper confidence

TABLE 3.1

Intersection–Union Test Results for Linifanib on QTcF

Regimens	Time Point (h)	QTcF Mean		Point[a] Estimate	95% Upper Confidence Bound
		Drug	Baseline		
Linifanib fasting regimen	0.5	421.8	423.9	−2.23	1.43
	1	422.0	423.1	−1.24	2.43
	2	422.1	421.4	0.57	4.24
	3	422.6	421.9	0.64	4.30
	4	418.1	422.4	−1.92	1.78
	6	415.8	419.9	−4.14	−0.47
	8	417.5	420.2	−2.82	0.85
	10	419.6	420.4	−0.58	3.12
	12	420.1	420.2	−0.16	3.50
	24	422.1	423.5	−1.53	2.14
Linifanib non-fasting regimen	0.5	419.8	423.9	−4.15	−0.48
	1	418.3	423.1	−4.89	−1.23
	2	417.1	421.4	−4.33	−0.67
	3	416.0	421.9	−6.03	−2.36
	4	413.8	422.4	−3.82	−0.12
	6	416.9	419.9	−3.05	0.61
	8	416.4	420.2	−3.87	−0.20
	10	417.2	419.4	−1.83	1.90
	12	417.3	418.9	−1.78	1.92
	24	421.0	422.4	−1.57	2.14

[a] Least square mean (ms) of change from baseline in QTcF interval (ΔQTcF).

bound for the drug effects for linifanib was 4.30 ms. These results are below the threshold of regulatory concern as indicated in ICH E14 Guidance for Industry.[4] It was therefore concluded that linifanib had no effect on cardiac repolarization.

The analysis was also performed with linifanib concentration as the drug exposure variable. The mixed effects model showed a linear relationship between changes in QTcF interval and linifanib concentration (Figure 3.1). The model estimated a slope of 0.01048, with a standard error of 0.006537 ($P = 0.1094$). This predicted a trend toward a change in the QTcF interval of 3.56 ms at a concentration of 0.34 ug/mL (the C_{max} at the MTD) and a 95% upper confidence bound of 7.2 ms. In addition to supporting the finding that linifanib does not significantly affect the QT interval, this model may provide useful predictions about the impact of other dosing regimens on QT prolongation.

The current study is one of a few to rigorously test the effect of an investigational drug on cardiac repolarization in patients with advanced tumors who are refractory to standard treatments. Analysis of the resulting data has concluded that linifanib does not pose a heightened risk for QTc prolongation in this refractory patient population. Despite a sample size of 24 subjects, the data had high operational and statistical precision as the 95% upper confidence bounds for mean differences from baseline were below the threshold of regulatory concern at all time points. Exposure–response modeling showed QTcF change was not significant at the maximum concentration for the MTD, which further supports a lack of QT prolongation with linifanib.

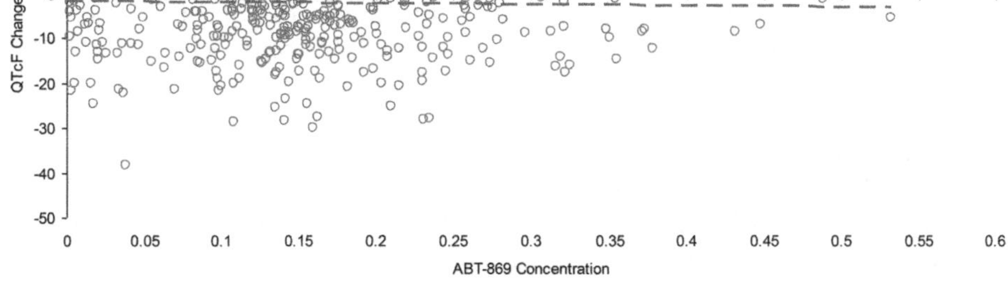

FIGURE 3.1
Linifanib concentration versus QTcF change from baseline (ΔQTcF).

3.2 The BE Study in Cancer Patients Using Group Sequential Design

3.2.1 Introduction

For pharmaceutical developers, it is important to compare the bioavailability of the drug from new formulations and/or strengths to that of formulations utilized in earlier phase clinical trials. For generic companies, a BE study is a necessary step in gaining regulatory approval and subsequent commercialization for the generic copy. If BE is established between a test small molecule agent and the reference formulation, it would be deemed unnecessary to conduct a large clinical study to demonstrate the equivalence in efficacy and safety. The BE criteria based on C_{max} and area under the curve (AUC) have been defined—the 90% CIs for the ratio of the test versus the reference formulations must be within 0.8 to 1.25. The BE criteria have been defined and accepted as a regulatory standard.[5] However, a BE study for oncology presents numerous challenges. In many cases, it is not feasible to administer cancer drug to healthy subjects like typical BE studies. Compared to those from healthy subjects confined in a phase 1 unit, the pharmacokinetic data in patients are less predictable as it is difficult to gain a complete control of study conditions. The enrollment in patients would be much slower and more dropouts would be anticipated. Due to these reasons, a group sequential crossover design is worth considering, because the study could be stopped early for either success or futility.[6] When a group sequential crossover BE study is well designed, compared to the gain in speed and resource savings, the price to pay would be small by expanding the CIs from 90% to slightly wider. By controlling the type I error within 5% for each side of the BE tests, the level of confidence (a figure between 90% and 95%) for the group sequential design would differ based on the predefined futility and success criteria. Here, the type I error for the upper one-sided test is the probability that the upper bound of a CI is less than 1.25 when the true ratio is 1.25 or greater. The same principle applies to the lower one-sided test. That is, the type I error for the lower one-sided test is the probability that the lower bound of a CI is greater than 0.80 when the true ratio is 0.80 or lower. If the data are analyzed only once at the end of the study (one look), the conventional type I error rate is set to 5% for each bound of the CI, and thus the confidence level is 90%. However, given a potential for two looks at the data, the CI will increase to a value that is greater than 90% at both stages to maintain the 5% type I error rate. The extent of the increase (e.g., to 92.7% from 90%) for the CI has to be evaluated based on the sample sizes and the futility/success criteria for both stages. If the results from Stage I do not indicate either success or futility, the trial will continue to Stage II. After the completion of Stage II, the data from both stages will be combined and analyzed.

An example of the results that gained regulatory approvals follows.

3.2.2 Methodology

This phase 1, open-label, multicenter study was conducted according to a four-period, group sequential, crossover design in subjects with solid tumors. The main objectives of the study were to assess the relative bioavailability of three new 40 mg capsule formulations of a drug. The study was planned as two stages, with a pharmacokinetic interim analysis conducted after the completion of Stage I. The study was to continue to Stage II only if results from Stage I interim analysis were unable to indicate bioequivalence success or futility.

Subjects were randomly assigned in equal numbers to receive four regimens of a single oral dose of 40 mg of veliparib capsules (Table 3.2) randomized through one of four sequence groups (Table 3.3). The regimens were supplied as four 10-mg capsules (current formulation, Regimen A), four 10-mg new capsules (new formulation, Regimen B), and one 40-mg capsule under fasting conditions (new strength Regimen C), under fasting conditions (Regimen C), and under non-fasting conditions (Regimen D). The study drug was administered in the morning on Study Day 1 of each period under fasting conditions in Regimen A, B, and C. Subjects receiving Regimen D were administered the dose of study drug 30 min after starting a high-fat breakfast. Serial blood samples were collected for 24 h after dosing in each period. Subjects remained at the study site and were supervised for approximately

TABLE 3.2

Veliparib Regimens Evaluated in the Study

Regimen	Description
A	Four 10-mg veliparib capsules (clinical) administered under fasting conditions.
B	Four 10-mg veliparib capsules (commercial) administered under fasting conditions.
C	One 40-mg veliparib capsule (commercial) administered under fasting conditions.
D	One 40-mg veliparib capsule (commercial) administered under non-fasting conditions.

TABLE 3.3

Planned Sequence Groups for Administration of Veliparib Regimens in the Study

Sequence	Number of Subjects		Veliparib Regimens			
Group	Stage I	Stage II*	Period 1	Period 2	Period 3	Period 4
I	5	4	A	B	C	D
II	5	4	B	D	A	C
III	5	4	C	A	D	B
IV	5	4	D	C	B	A

* Stage II of this study was not conducted.

16 h in each study period. Subjects returned to the center for the Study Day 2 pharmacokinetic sample.

Twenty subjects were planned for the enrollment in Stage I; on the basis of the pharmacokinetic interim analysis, an additional 16 subjects were to be enrolled in Stage II. The two-stage, group sequential design was used to offer an early opportunity to evaluate the bioavailability of the test formulations. Enrollment for Stage I preceded until 20 subjects had completed all four periods of the assigned sequences. After the completion of Stage I and depending on results from the statistical analysis on the data collected from these Stage I subjects, the study would stop if the results were sufficiently convincing. If additional data were required, the study would have continued with enrollment into Stage II until 16 additional subjects had completed all four periods of their assigned sequences in Stage II. If the study had continued through Stage II, subjects from both stages would have been included in the final statistical evaluation.

Appropriate statistical adjustments were made to protect against inflation of the type I error rate due to the potential for two looks at the pharmacokinetic data (after Stage I and potentially after Stage II). Type I error is defined as falsely rejecting the null hypothesis when the null hypothesis is true. Here, the type I error for the upper one-sided test is the probability that the upper bound of a CI is less than 1.25 when the true ratio is 1.25 or greater. The same principle applies to the lower one-sided test. That is, the type I error for the lower one-sided test is the probability that the lower bound of a CI is greater than 0.80 when the true ratio is 0.80 or lower.

If the data are analyzed only once at the end of the study (one look), the conventional type I error rate is set to 5% for each bound of the CI, and thus the confidence level is 90%. For a two-stage group sequential BE study, the CI has to be adjusted to a level that is greater than 90% for both stages to maintain the 5% type I error rate. For this particular example, the CI was raised to 92.7% (instead of 90%) at both stages. In the simulations, various figures from 90% to 95% for CI were evaluated within the framework of the design until the overall type I error rate fell under 5%, using the planned study sizes for both stages and the stopping rule for futility after Stage I. Therefore, when the true ratio is 1.25 (the test formulation is not bioequivalent to the reference formulation), the chance of observing an upper bound of the 92.7% CI that is less than 1.25 (rejecting the null hypothesis) in Stage I or Stage II is maintained within 5%.

Two potential outcomes will correspond to sufficiently convincing results from Stage I and trigger termination of the study. In the successful outcome, the BE criteria are met using the 92.7% CIs obtained from the Stage I data. In the futile outcome, the data indicate that the test regimen is clearly not similar to the reference. Futility at Stage I is defined as not meeting the BE criteria with 92.7% CI and the lower bound of the 92.7% CI >1.069. This criterion was chosen such that when the ratio is 1.25 (the test formulation is not bioequivalent to the reference formulation), the chance of terminating the study at Stage I due to futility is at least 55%. If the results from Stage I do not indicate either success or futility, the trial will continue to Stage II. After the completion of Stage II, the data from both stages will be combined, analyzed, and the 92.7% CI will be calculated.

The study size consideration was based on the primary comparison of the test Regimen B to the reference Regimen A within the modeling framework. The probability of rejecting either one-sided null hypothesis (that the ratio is not greater than 0.80 or that the ratio is not less than 1.25) using the 92.7% CI was computed assuming the within-subject variability (as estimated by the crossover analysis of variance mean square error or MSE term from a previous veliparib study) of 0.06 for the natural logarithm of C_{max}. The variability for AUC is expected to be similar.

The power calculations were carried out using 10,000 Monte Carlo simulations for 20 and 36 subjects for Stage I and the combination of Stages I and II, respectively. The term "success," as opposed to futility, is used when the BE criteria are met. Assuming the true ratio of 1.05, the overall power (successfully rejecting the null hypothesis at stage I or the combination of Stages I and II) is 89.6%, the probability of stopping after Stage I due to success or futility is 64% and 1.5%, respectively. In the Monte Carlo simulations, the underlying population for C_{max} was assumed to follow the log-normal probability distribution. The critical *t*-value with the appropriate degree of freedom was used for the sampling distribution of the mean difference on the natural logarithmic scale. If the true ratio is 1.05, the study will provide approximately 64% power for meeting the BE criteria in Stage I. As the true ratio shifts from 1.05 toward 1, the power would become greater.

Under the null hypothesis where the true ratio is 1.25, the overall type I error rate is maintained below 5% based on 20,000 simulations (average rate: 4.91%) given this study design. The chance of stopping after Stage I due to futility is 55.2%.

The study design is illustrated in Figure 3.2.

A linear mixed effects analysis was performed for T_{max}, elimination rate constant β, and the natural logarithms of C_{max}, AUC_t, and AUC_{inf}. The model accounted for within and between subject variability and included effects for sequence, period, and regimen. The model employed compound-symmetry variance-covariance structure among regimens. The Kenward–Roger approximation was used to assess the degrees of freedom. Within the linear mixed effects model framework, four pairs of regimens were compared by a test with a significance level of 0.05— Regimen B versus A, Regimen C versus A, Regimen C versus B (to assess BE), and Regimen D versus C (to characterize the effect of a high-fat meal on bioavailability).

The relative bioavailability between each pair was assessed by the two one-sided tests procedure via 92.7% CIs obtained from the analyses of the natural logarithms of C_{max} and AUC. To control the overall type I error under 5%, a 92.7% CI was computed instead of the typical 90% in the testing of BE of any pharmacokinetic parameter between any two regimens to maintain

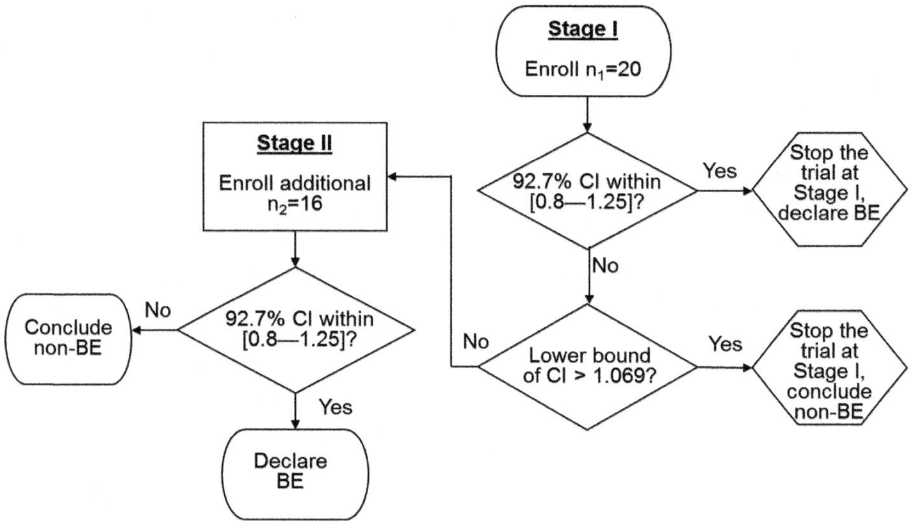

FIGURE 3.2
Two-stage group sequence design.

the overall type I error within 5% using the planned study sizes for both stages and the stopping rule for futility after Stage I. The CIs were obtained by exponentiation of the endpoints of confidence intervals for the difference of mean logarithms obtained within the framework of the model. The BE between each pair was concluded if the 92.7% CIs from the analyses of the natural logarithms of AUC and C_{max} were within the 0.80–1.25 range. The point estimates of the relative bioavailability (i.e., the ratio of the geometric means) were likewise obtained by exponentiation of the least squares estimate of the difference of mean logarithms and the population central value for each regimen was estimated by exponentiation of the least squares mean for the logarithm.

3.2.3 Results and Conclusion

In an effort to ensure that a total of 20 subjects had completed all four periods for the Stage I analysis, enrolment was allowed to continue beyond the first 20 subjects. A total of 27 subjects were enrolled into Stage I and 23 subjects completed at least two periods of the study. The first 20 subjects (based on date and time of the first dose) who completed all four periods and provided evaluable pharmacokinetic data from all four periods were included in the primary statistical analysis of pharmacokinetic parameters for Stage I, as prespecified in the study protocol. For the 20 subjects included in the statistical analysis (4 males and 16 females), the mean age was 55.4 years (range = 29–79 years), the mean weight was 70.8 kg (range = 52–88 kg), and the mean height was 165 cm (range = 140–185 cm). A secondary statistical analysis was conducted for Stage I that included all subjects ($N = 23$) that completed at least two periods of the study. Results from the secondary analysis were similar to the primary analysis. Stage I interim analysis provided evidence for BE across the different formulations and the study was considered complete; Stage II was not conducted.

The mean ± standard deviation (SD) pharmacokinetic parameters of veliparib after administration of each of the four regimens to subjects with solid tumors are presented in Table 3.4. Period and sequence effects were not statistically significant for any of the tested pharmacokinetic parameters, as all p-values for the test on period and sequence effects were ≥0.544 and 0.450, respectively. Mean veliparib plasma concentration–time profiles following the single oral doses of Regimens A, B, and C are presented in Figure 3.3. The test statistics for the regimen effect for T_{max}, C_{max}, and β were not statistically significant ($P < 0.05$). The central values for AUC_t and AUC_{inf} for Regimen B (four 10-mg new formulation, fasting) were statistically significantly higher ($P = 0.002$ and $P = 0.003$, respectively) than those for the reference Regimen A (four 10-mg current formulation, fasting). The central values for AUC_t and AUC_{inf} for Regimen C (one 40-mg strength of veliparib commercial capsule new formulation, fasting) were statistically significantly lower than those for Regimen B ($P < 0.001$). There was no statistically significant difference ($P > 0.05$) between Regimen C (40-mg veliparib commercial capsules, fasting) and Regimen A in AUC_t and AUC_{inf}.

The 92.7% CIs for evaluating BE and the corresponding point estimates from the analysis of log-transformed C_{max}, AUC_t, and AUC_{inf} for comparisons of veliparib regimens are shown in Table 3.5. Regimen A, B, and C were bioequivalent. All 92.7% CIs for evaluating the BE of Regimens A, B, and C for C_{max}, AUC_t, and AUC_{inf} of veliparib were contained within the 0.80–1.25 range.

TABLE 3.4

Summary of Veliparib Pharmacokinetic Parameters (Mean ± SD)

Pharmacokinetic Parameters	(units)	40 mg Veliparib ($N = 20$)			
		A: Four 10-mg Clinical Capsules Fasting	B: Four 10-mg Commercial Capsules Fasting	C: One 40-mg Commercial Capsule Fasting	D: One 40-mg Commercial Capsule Non–Fasting
T_{max}	(h)	1.2 ± 0.8	1.2 ± 0.7	1.3 ± 0.9	2.5 ± 1.1
C_{max}	(μg/mL)	0.36 ± 0.13	0.37 ± 0.12	0.34 ± 0.12	0.28 ± 0.09
AUC_t	(μg·h/mL)	2.23 ± 0.82	2.45 ± 0.93	2.24 ± 0.98	2.14 ± 0.80
AUC_{inf}	(μg·h/mL)	2.43 ± 1.07	2.65 ± 1.17	2.45 ± 1.24	2.35 ± 1.06
$t_{½}$[a]	(h)	5.95 ± 1.26	5.83 ± 1.23	5.83 ± 1.31	5.85 ± 1.36
CL/F[b]	(L/h)	19.0 ± 7.36	17.3 ± 6.41	19.5 ± 7.66	19.7 ± 7.51

[a] Harmonic mean ± pseudo-standard deviation; evaluations of $t_{½}$ were based on statistical tests for λ.

[b] Parameter was not tested statistically.

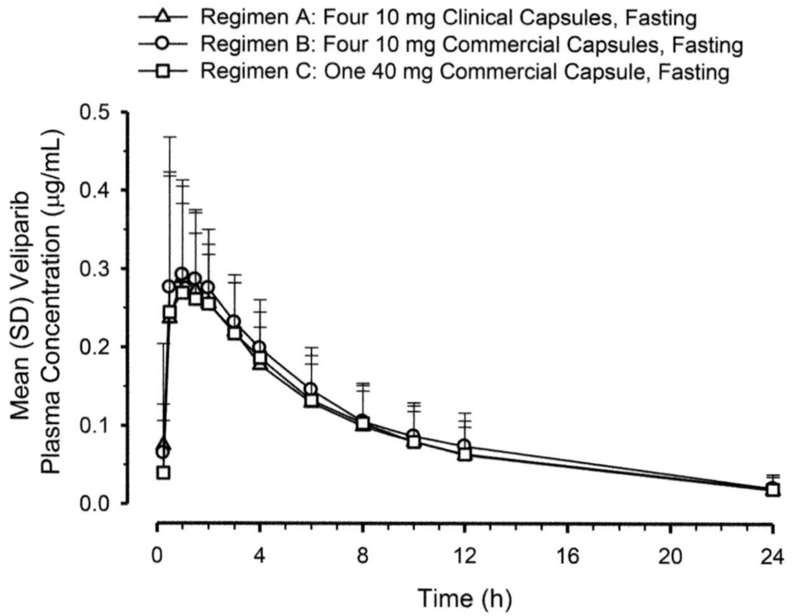

FIGURE 3.3
Veliparib mean (+SD) plasma concentration-time profiles following oral administration of Veliparib.

TABLE 3.5
Relative Bioavailability and 92.7% CIs for the BE Assessment

Regimens Test vs. Reference	Pharmacokinetic Parameter	Central Value[a]		Relative Bioavailability	
		Test	Reference	Point Estimate[b]	92.7% CI
B vs. A	C_{max}	0.348	0.337	1.031	0.925–1.150
	AUC_t	2.306	2.106	1.095	1.040–1.153
	AUC_{inf}	2.463	2.255	1.093	1.037–1.152
C vs. B	C_{max}	0.322	0.348	0.927	0.831–1.033
	AUC_t	2.078	2.306	0.901	0.856–0.949
	AUC_{inf}	2.223	2.463	0.902	0.856–0.951
D vs. C	C_{max}	0.266	0.322	0.827	0.741–0.922
	AUC_t	2.011	2.078	0.968	0.919–1.019
	AUC_{inf}	2.174	2.223	0.978	0.928–1.031
C vs. A	C_{max}	0.322	0.337	0.956	0.857–1.066
	AUC_t	2.078	2.106	0.987	0.937–1.039
	AUC_{inf}	2.223	2.255	0.986	0.935–1.039

[a] Antilogarithm of the least squares means for logarithms.
[b] Antilogarithm of the difference (test minus reference) of the least squares means for logarithm.

The group sequential design was efficient in this case, as the 92.7% CIs are only slightly wider than those of the conventional 90%, while the study was stopped early for success.

3.3 Exposure-Adjusted Continual Reassessment Method for Dose-Finding Studies

3.3.1 Introduction

In phase 1 studies, the most important primary objective is to find the MTD. Drug exposure and toxicity events are the two major components required for the characterization of MTD. It has often been assumed in the literature as well as in clinical practice, as a simplified approach, that the toxicity outcome can be observed before a given time *T*, and the assigned dose level would represent the drug exposure leading to the outcome of with or without toxicity before time *T*. Consequently, many phase 1 oncology dose-finding designs, including the traditional 3 + 3 fixed designs and various versions of adaptive continual reassessment methods (CRM)[7] have been operated under a set of distinct cohorts of patients with a predefined observational period (e.g., the first cycle) for tracking the toxicity outcomes. The dose-escalation decisions have been made periodically, requiring all the patients within the cohort of the assigned dose to be enrolled and followed up until crossing the finish line of the observational period.

In addition to the operational restrictions, strong clinical and statistical assumptions are made for those conventional dose escalation studies including fixed and adaptive designs—the observational period is chosen properly such that the intended toxicity incidence would follow the stochastic process according to the underlying population true incidence rate. Moreover, the expected time of onset for dose-related toxicity is assumed to be the same across different patients and all dose levels considered in the study. While there might be situations where it would be possible to measure the two required components—drug exposure and toxicity outcome—with an approximation by fixing the observational period and using the assigned dose level, the strong clinical and statistical assumptions rarely hold. The duration for the observational period is often set up based on the assumed hematologic recovery period, more subjectively on the assumed toxicities that are expected, or based purely on practicality; otherwise, if a study stretches the observational period to capture delayed-onset toxicities, the dose-finding process will be substantially delayed before moving on to the next cohort. As a result, the conventional dose-escalation designs that treat many patients at subtherapeutic doses unnecessarily prolong the time of studies, are often inaccurate in determining true toxicity rates, and rarely allow estimation of clinical response at doses to be used in phase 2 studies. These designs also have the disadvantage of periodic closures and lengthy accrual time and often lose momentum because of the episodic nature of accrual.[8] The operational and clinical challenges, include major drawbacks such as 1) the time to the toxicity event is not accounted for, 2) the extent of drug exposure leading to the onset of toxicity is not measured correctly, and 3) delayed-onset toxicities past the cutoff observation period are not captured. The improvements should be made to attain more accurate information on the extent of exposure and the time to event, with a more dynamic enrolment to facilitate better decision-making at the early phase, thereby increasing the probability of success in treating patients.

To address the major drawbacks as described earlier, statistical methodology has been proposed in the literature including using sequential designs for phase 1 clinical trials with late-onset toxicities (TITE-CRM) by Ying Kuen Cheung and Rick Chappell[9] via the maximum likelihood approach, and Bayesian approach by Suyu Liu and Jing Ning[10] for drug combination trials with delayed toxicities. The objective of our research is to address the major drawbacks of the conventional designs by proposing a robust methodology that is readily implementable in real clinical practice. Furthermore, the operational hurdle of periodic closures is overcome by being able to enroll patients in a staggered fashion.

3.3.2 Methodology

The EACRM assumes continuous enrollment of patients/subjects with a calculation of the estimated MTD for each subject enrolled at the corresponding time point. An accelerated failure time (AFT) model with dose level as the covariate will be employed to characterize the time to dose-limiting toxicity (DLT). The proposed AFT model is:

$$\log(T) = \alpha + \beta D + \sigma\epsilon,$$

where D is the dose level and T is the time to DLT. The AFT model assumes a linear relationship between the mean of the logarithm of time to DLT and dose level as α and β denote the intercept and slope, respectively.[8] Moreover, σ is a positive parameter that controls the variability of the model and ϵ denotes the error term. In this paper, we assume that T follows either a log-Normal or a Weibull distribution. More specifically, under the log-Normal model, $T \sim \text{LN}(\alpha + \beta D, \sigma^2)$ and $\epsilon \sim N(0,1)$ and the Weibull model, $T \sim W(\sigma^{-1}, e^{\alpha+\beta D})$ and ϵ follows a standard extreme value distribution with density function $f_\epsilon(v) = e^{v-e^{v}}$.

As an incorporation of the time-to-event information, let δ be the indicator of DLT ($\delta = 1$ for DLT) and let w denote the weight of an observation. Essentially, the weight factor will control the contribution to the likelihood function from each data point during the estimation process. Given a set of full data $\{(T_i, \delta_i, D_i, w_i)\}_{i=1}^{n}$ and the corresponding density function *f*, the problem can be well characterized under the framework of survival analysis. The likelihood function is written as:

$$L(T \mid \alpha, \beta, \sigma) = \prod_{i:\delta_i=1} \left[f(T_i \mid \alpha + \beta D_i, \sigma) \right]^{w_i} \cdot \prod_{i:\delta_i=0} \left[1 - F(T_i \mid \alpha + \beta D_i, \sigma) \right]^{w_i}.$$

A frequentist approach based on maximum likelihood method with the Newton–Raphson algorithm will be utilized for the model estimation process. To assign the dose level to the next subject entering our trial, predictions of time to DLT are made based on all m possible dose levels $\{d_j : d_0 + jd; j = 1, \ldots, m\}$ with $d_0$mg starting dose and d mg increment.

$$D_{n+1} = \max\left\{ d_j : \hat{T}_{1/3}(d_j) \geq L; j = 1, \ldots, m \right\}, \tag{3.1}$$

where L is a prespecified toxicity assessment period of study and $\hat{T}_{1/3}(D)$ indicates that we are predicting the 1/3 quantile of the time to DLT for the new dose level as it is the usual threshold for DLT rate allowed. Once the estimated parameters, $\hat{\alpha}$, $\hat{\beta}$, and $\hat{\sigma}$ are obtained, we can update the estimation of the time-dose curve given the derived formula as follows: for the log-Normal model, $\hat{T}_{1/3}(D) = e^{\hat{\alpha}+\hat{\beta}D-0.431\hat{\sigma}}$; for the Weibull model, $\hat{T}_{1/3}(D) = e^{\hat{\alpha}+\hat{\beta}D-0.903\hat{\sigma}}$. Note that the estimates $\hat{\alpha}$, $\hat{\beta}$, and $\hat{\sigma}$ are different under two models.

As mentioned previously, the model we proposed is able to utilize not only the toxicity events but also the time-to-event information by specifying appropriate time responses $\{T_i\}_{i=1}^{n}$ and weights $\{w_i\}_{i=1}^{n}$ in the AFT model. Although there is no unique mathematical approach for the weights, it is natural and practical to make some basic assumptions about them: 1) Given a specific time point during the trial, a non-DLT subject with longer survival period (e.g., 9 weeks without having a DLT) is expected to have a lower probability of a DLT occurrence than one with shorter survival period (e.g., 2 weeks without having a DLT) and hence higher weight of surviving entire toxicity assessment period without DLT occurrence. 2) In general, the weight should be an increasing function of observed time t_0 taking values in [0, 1]. A weight of 1 indicates that the information from that individual is fully used in the model.

A good candidate for the weight is the conditional probability of completion or no DLT, given the observed time. For example, if the duration of the observation period is L weeks long and t_0 is the observed time, then the conditional probability is given by $P(T > L \mid T > t_0)$. It will be generic if we want the weights to be independent of the distribution of T, since the true distribution may not be known in the real case. However, to calculate the weights, we have to assume a specific distribution. And we point out that a distribution with constant hazards will be sufficient when the subject is on a particular dose level over the entire toxicity assessment period. Throughout this section, we let T be the time to DLT with mean time to DLT λ and assume $T \mid \lambda \sim \text{Exp}(\lambda)$ with density function, which is a special case of Weibull distribution with shape parameter value of 1 given by

$$f_T(t) = \lambda e^{-\lambda t},\ t \geq 0.$$

Note that this would assume constant hazard of observing DLT at each dose level. Under the Bayesian framework, it is natural to consider a Gamma prior for λ, that is, $\lambda \sim \text{Gamma}(a, b)$ with shape parameter a and rate parameter b.

It follows that the posterior distribution for λ remains to be a Gamma distribution: $\lambda \mid t \sim \text{Gamma}(a+1, b+t)$. Meanwhile, recall that we allow at most 1/3 DLT rate when seeking the MTD, which gives us a restriction between λ and the duration of the observation period, L:

$$P(T < L \mid \lambda) = 1 - e^{-L\lambda} = 1/3 \Rightarrow \lambda = \frac{1}{L}\log(3/2).$$

Then, under an approximate relationship, we have

$$E(\lambda) = \frac{a}{b} \approx \lambda \Rightarrow a = \frac{b}{L}\log(3/2).$$

Given all the information on distributions and parameters, now consider

$$E(\lambda \mid T = t_0) = \frac{a+1}{b+t_0} = \frac{b\log(3/2)/L + 1}{b+t_0} = \lambda^{*}.$$

If we fix $\lambda = \lambda^{*}$, then for $0 < t_0 < L$, the probability of completing the toxicity assessment period without DLT is

$$p^{*}(t_0) = P(T > L \mid T > t_0) = \frac{P(T > L)}{P(T > t_0)} = e^{-\lambda^{*}(L - t_0)}.$$

Moreover, it can be shown that $T \mid t_0 < T < L$ follows a truncated exponential distribution with conditional expectation

$$E(T \mid t_0) = E(T \mid t_0 < T < L) = \int_{t_0}^{L} \frac{\lambda^{*} t e^{-\lambda^{*} t}}{e^{-\lambda^{*} t_0} - e^{-\lambda^{*} L}}\,dt = \frac{F_\Gamma(L \mid 2, \lambda^{*}) - F_\Gamma(t_0 \mid 2, \lambda^{*})}{\lambda^{*}\left(e^{-\lambda^{*} t_0} - e^{-\lambda^{*} L}\right)},$$

where $F_\Gamma(\cdot \mid 2, \lambda^{*})$ is the cumulative distribution function of $\text{Gamma}(2, \lambda^{*})$.

Given the derivation of all the relevant probabilities and distributions as shown, the response and weight for each subject are presented in Table 3.6.

On the basis of the introduction to our model as mentioned earlier, at each time point that a new subject enters the trial, MTD will be reestimated based

TABLE 3.6

Specification of Response and its Weight in Model

Progress of a Subject in Trial	Response (T_i)	Weight (w_i)
Completed without DLT	L	1
Observed with DLT	t_{DLT}	1
In Progress and $t_0 + E(T \mid t_0) \geq L$	L	$p^*(t_0)$
In Progress and $t_0 + E(T \mid t_0) < L$	$t_0 + E(T \mid t_0)$	$1 - p^*(t_0)$

on all available observations using a parametric survival regression model. Then a simple algorithm can be provided as follows, assuming that at most n subjects are recruited for the study and the time of enrollment follows a certain distribution, for example, an exponential distribution with rate τ.

First, allow three subjects to go through the entire trial process with either completion or DLT as the outcomes and check certain futility criteria (Table 3.7).

Starting from the fourth subject, proceed iteratively for $3 \leq k \leq n-1$:

When the $(k+1)$-th subject enters the trial, determine the time on the toxicity assessment period, DLT status, and corresponding weight for all k existing subjects: $(T_1, \delta_1, w_1), \ldots, (T_k, \delta_k, w_k)$.

Drop all non-DLT observations that have small exposures, for example, less than 10% out of the entire toxicity assessment period.

Perform survival regression based on the AFT model. Use effective data collected from the given steps.

Obtain the 1/3 quantile predictions for time to DLT for all dose levels $\{d_j\}_{j=1}^{m}$ and assign proper dose level D_{k+1} to the $(k+1)$-th subject based on formula (3.1).

Determine if MTD is achieved based on the clinically not significant change in predicted MTD and end the iteration if necessary.

Verify the estimated MTD and collect summary statistics for time and dose variables.

Note that the futility criteria and conditions for MTD attainment may vary by specific studies. However, some general guidelines are highly desirable. For instance, a negative sign of the estimated slope for dose, β, is expected in each iteration and some convergence check for the dose assignment will be necessary when seeking the MTD.

TABLE 3.7

Parameterization and Distribution Matrix

Prior Distribution Used for Weight Derivation	Distribution for Time to DLT is Log-Normal	Distribution for Time to DLT is Weibull
Gamma(a, b)	LN1	W1
Gamma(aD, b)	LN2	W2
Gamma(a, b/D)	LN3	W3

TABLE 3.8

Specification of True Distribution

Log-Normal Distribution: $T \sim \text{LN}\left(\alpha_{\text{LN}} + \beta_{\text{LN}} D, \sigma_{\text{LN}}^2\right)$		
Parameter\Targeted Dose	**120 mg**	**70 mg**
α_{LN}	2.6615	2.5500
β_{LN}	–0.0022	–0.0022
σ_{LN}	0.2239	0.2239
Weibull Distribution: $T \sim W\left(\sigma_W^{-1}, e^{\alpha_W + \beta_W D}\right)$		
Parameter\Targeted Dose	**120 mg**	**70 mg**
α_W	2.7820	2.8052
β_W	–0.0022	–0.0022
σ_W	0.2379	0.3857

This methodology was utilized in locally advanced rectal cancer study that administered the investigational drug in combination with chemotherapy and radiation therapy. The toxicity assessment period was 8 weeks. The dose range planned to be investigated was 20–400 mg twice daily (BID), with an anticipated MTD at 250 mg BID (Table 3.8).

We note that our exposure-adjusted design provides a more accurate prediction of MTD. Also, the prediction clearly indicates that the expected survival time *E*(*T*) decreases as the dose level *D* increases. But the previous designs assume no association between the expected time to DLT, *E*(*T*), and dose *D*, since $E(T) = E(1/\lambda) = b/(a-1)$. Therefore, a possible re-parameterization for λ is given by

$$E(T) = \frac{b}{a-1} g(D),$$

which can allow such negative trend of the time–dose curve, where *g*(*D*) is a monotonically decreasing, positive function of dose *D*. Two simple but straightforward choices are 1) $\lambda \sim \text{Gamma}(\text{aD}, b)$ with $E(T) = \dfrac{b}{\text{aD} - 1}$ and 2) $\lambda \sim \text{Gamma}(a, b/D)$ with $E(T) = \dfrac{b}{(a-1)D}$. Hence, we will consider both parameterizations of λ along with the original design that $\lambda \sim \text{Gamma}(a, b)$ (Table 3.9).

Note that due to the maximum of 1/3 DLT rate allowed, we anticipate similar restrictions on hyper-parameters *a* and *b* for both re-parameterizations of λ, as specified earlier. However, since the dose level is involved, such restrictions can be only achieved at a given "targeted" dose level D_0, which leads to $a = \dfrac{\log(3/2)}{L} \cdot \dfrac{b}{D_0}$. This relationship holds for both cases. Once D_0 is specified, which simply could be an assumed MTD, there will be only

TABLE 3.9

Pseudo-Data Assignment

Observation #/Variable	Time (Weeks)	DLT Status (1 = Yes)	Dose (mg)	Weight
1	10	0	60	0.09
2	8	1	60	0.01
3	10	0	120	0.07
4	8	1	120	0.03
5	10	0	200	0.04
6	8	1	200	0.06

one free hyper-parameter, say, b. Then, as the rate parameter in Gamma distribution, b can be chosen as any positive constant. However, recall that $E(T)=\frac{b}{\text{aD}-1}$ for the first case and $E(T)=\frac{b}{(a-1)D}$ for the second one. To ensure that $E(T)>0$ for all possible dose levels starting from some initial dose d_0, we need $b>\frac{\text{LD}_0}{d_0\log(3/2)}$ for the first case and $b>\frac{\text{LD}_0}{\log(3/2)}$ for the second. Therefore, generally, the minimum value for b in the latter case is d_0 times the one in the former case.

We conducted the simulations to study the performance of the proposed EACRM design described in Section 3.2. Depending on different assumptions on the true distribution of the time to DLT and the time–dose structure (in terms of parameterizations of λ), we consider the following six cases:

We compare our six cases with the traditional 3 + 3 design and EACRM setting without using weights. For each case, we run 1,000 simulations based on two targeted MTDs—120 mg and 70 mg. The investigated dose range is 10–250 mg and the toxicity assessment period is set to be 10 weeks. The maximum number of enrolled subjects is 40 for each trial (simulation). The arbitrary enrollment rate $\tau = 1/4$ leads to an average of 4 weeks waiting time between two consecutive subjects. We also assume the rate parameter for Gamma, $b = 500$ for LN1, LN2, W1, W2, and $b = 3{,}000$ for LN3 and W3 to guarantee that the probability of observing DLT within the toxicity assessment period to be not greater than 33% and $E(T)>0$. If greater than 33% DLT rate is observed at the first tested dose level , the study is stopped for futility. The iteration of the algorithm is stopped if the change in predicted MTD is not clinically significant, that is, less than 10% increment from the current dose level.

The parameters of true distributions that we choose are shown in the following table.

The parameters are specified in a way that: 1) they result in the corresponding targeted MTD; 2) the slope coefficients of dose remain the same, and 3) all the other parameters are comparable under different targeted doses and distributions.

During the early stage of simulation, as subjects start to enter into a trial, the sample size may be small (e.g., 3–5), which usually results in a failure in the convergence of the estimation under survival regression. Hence, it is necessary to add a small number of pseudo-data into the regression as early observations. These pseudo data will be fixed throughout the study and will help in the model fitting process by solving convergence issues encountered during the early stage of the study. Appropriate weights will be assigned to them to reflect only a small degree of certainty. The pseudo-data we used are shown in Table 3.9.

Some general guidelines for pseudo-data selection can be described as follows:

1. Consider three dose levels in the lower, middle, and upper spectrum of the dose range to be investigated.
2. At each selected dose level in step 1, consider two data points, one with DLT occurring close to the end of toxicity assessment period and the other without DLT at the end of toxicity assessment period.
3. Assign a very small weight (≤0.1) to those six data points. Also, consider the possibility of having a DLT event at a selected dose level based on prior assumptions. For example, the possibility of a DLT event at a lower dose level is less compared to the possibility of a DLT event at a higher dose level.

A sensitivity analysis was carried out by altering the pseudo-data points generated using the above guidelines. We point out that the pseudo-data will not have a notable impact on the final simulation results. In real practice, it is also very unlikely that the MTD will be achieved based on only a few data points.

3.3.3 Results and Conclusion

We simulated all six cases for EACRM (LN1-LN3, W1-W3), two cases for EACRM without weights (LN0 and W0), as well as the 3 + 3 design (3 + 3) under both 120-mg and 70-mg targeted doses. The summary statistics are listed in Table 3.10 for 120-mg targeted dose. The 25%, 50%, and 75% label denotes the corresponding quartiles of the distribution of variables including the median.

Figure 3.4 summarizes and visualizes the simulation process of six cases for EACRM under the 120-mg targeted MTD. In each plot, we show the true dose–toxicity curve as well as the distribution of a particular dose selected as MTD over 1,000 simulations.

On the basis of the simulation results, we claim some clear advantages of our proposed EACRM over the traditional 3 + 3 or standard survival regression model. First, by utilizing the DLT information as well as time on the study, the EACRM gives a more accurate estimate of MTD than the 3 + 3 in general. Such improvement of accuracy becomes more significant as the targeted (true) MTD increases as the distribution of the predicted MTD becomes more concentrated in terms of the variance and quantiles. It also allows for a more dynamic enrolment of subjects, facilitates better decision-making,

TABLE 3.10

Summary Statistics for Simulations Under Targeted Dose 120 mg

Case\	MTD (mg)			Trial Size			Trial Duration (weeks)			Med.
Stats.	25%	50%	75%	25%	50%	75%	25%	50%	75%	DLT (%)
LN1	90	110	130	20	23	28	82.3	96.9	114.1	26.7
W1	80	110	140	19	24	29	82.3	99.7	118.2	29.2
LN2	90	110	130	19	23	28	81.7	96.0	115.4	26.7
W2	80	110	140	20	24	29	82.8	100.4	118.8	28.6
LN3	90	110	130	19	23	28	80.6	97.2	115.4	26.7
W3	80	110	132.5	19	23	28	80.7	97.6	116.3	27.3
LN0	80	100	120	21	24	28	87.8	102.4	118.3	21.7
W0	70	100	120	20	24	28	81.5	99.7	120.0	24
3+3	40	90	120	15	24	30	90.0	144.0	180.0	21.4

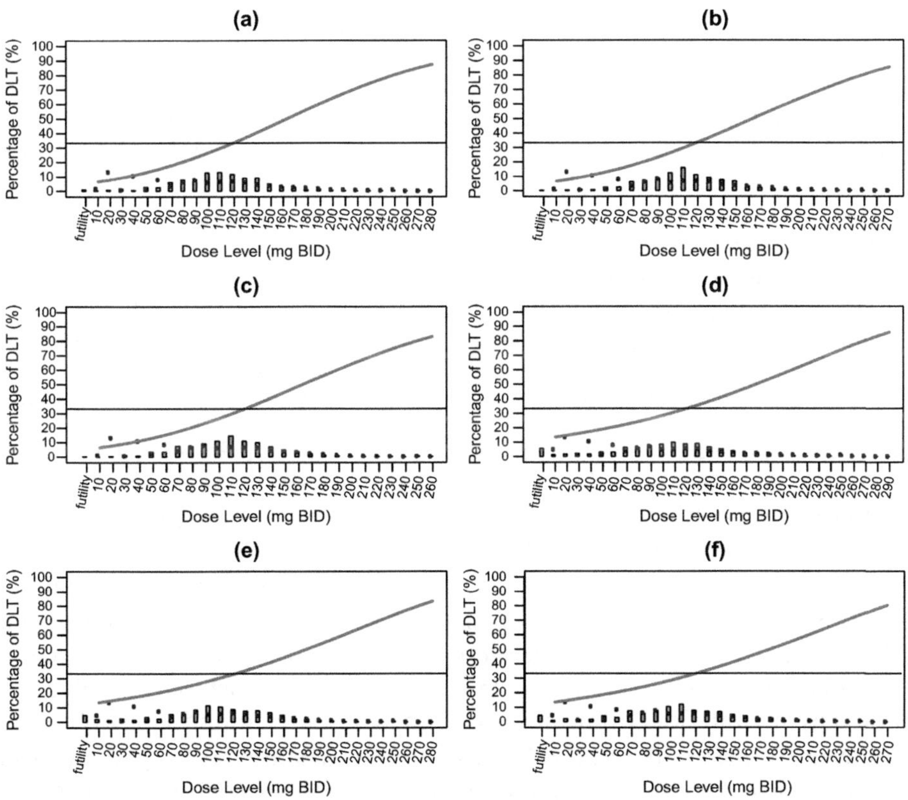

FIGURE 3.4

Plots for targeted MTD 120 mg: (a) Case LN1, (b) Case LN2, (c) Case LN3, (d) Case W1, (e) Case W2, and (f) Case W3.

thus requiring shorter duration and potentially fewer subjects for a study. Meanwhile, the AFT model with weights depending on dose levels provides both high flexibility and efficiency in modeling, and the combination of frequentist approach for model estimation and Bayesian approach for weight determination shows more reasonable predictions for MTD.

When comparing the results from different distributions, we find that the Weibull distribution demonstrates more variability when determining the MTD than the log-Normal distribution, although it may require a shorter duration of the study. The EACRM keeps underestimating the true MTD slightly due to its conservative nature.

Although EACRM provided a satisfactory performance in terms of dose finding, it is commonly agreed among clinicians and biostatisticians that, as an adaptive design, the CRMs offer more aggressive dose escalation, which may raise a notable safety concern.[7] Therefore, certain appropriate stopping criteria may be applied when selecting the MTD. Moreover, to handle a method with such a high flexibility in modeling, a good knowledge of both clinical trial and statistics will be essential. In practice, for first-in-human studies that employ the EACRM, we have identified specific measures to ensure subject safety: 1) the first subject enrolled should complete the entire observation period prior to any dose escalations, 2) at the time of a DLT, any subject that enrolled at higher dose levels should have the option to reduce the current dose dependent on the toxicity observed, 3) some staggering of subject enrolment is required. Thus it has been proved that in the event of very aggressive enrolment, no more than six subjects can be enrolled at the same dose level.

We also want to point out that there is always room for improvement regarding our proposed models and methods. For instance, a straightforward generalization of the time–dose relationship can be made by developing more complicated but flexible priors on λ when deriving the weights such as $\lambda \sim \text{Gamma}(a_0 + a_1 D, b)$ or $\lambda \sim \text{Gamma}\left(a, \frac{b_1}{b_0 + D}\right)$. By introducing the intercept term, we obtain a full linear function of dose level $\boldsymbol{D}$, which is able to fit a variety of decreasing curves that may be necessary since the pattern of time–dose curves can be more moderate as the predicted MTD goes up. Another generalization is applicable on the distribution of T. When specifying the weights we consider an exponential distribution $T \sim \text{Exp}(\lambda)$ resulting in a constant hazard, which can be extended to a Weibull distribution, $T \sim W(K, \lambda)$ with more general hazard given the shape parameter K and rate parameter λ. Then, to obtain an appropriate posterior distribution, one may assume less informative Gamma priors for K and λ or even non-informative priors like $\pi(\theta) \propto 1$ or $\pi(\theta) \propto 1/\theta$, where θ is any parameter of interest. However, the corresponding posterior distributions have no known closed forms. Thus, some sampling techniques for Bayesian inference such as the Markov Chain Monte Carlo method may be needed for obtaining the posteriors and will be based on conditional distributions.

3.4 Using Exposure-Safety Response Models for Dose Selection of the Late Phase Pivotal Study

3.4.1 Introduction

For virtually any compound, choosing the right dose or dosing regimen for balancing safety and efficacy is crucial for the probability of success. In conventional drug development process, the dose tested in the late phase registration study is commonly selected based on promising results(s) given by the same dose and similar indication and patient population from the early phase. The early phase outcomes in the oncology therapeutic area, however, are often confounded by numerous dosing regimens in a variety of populations. The dosing regimens could include different dosage strengths (e.g., 10 mg versus 400 mg), dosing frequencies (e.g., BID) versus once daily (QD)), fixed or variable regimens (e.g., 400 mg versus 5 mg/kg), formulations (e.g., solid dosage form versus liquid), number and length of cycles, dosing interruptions, concurrent medications, diets, and so on. Therefore, it is of value to take advantage of pharmacokinetic exposure to correlate with the safety or efficacy outcomes. The following example provides an analysis to identify the dose/dosing regimen for the phase 3 study.

3.4.2 Methodology

An exposure–response (safety) analysis was performed for patients enrolled in one phase 1 and three phase 2 monotherapy studies conducted internationally. The mean body weight was 68 kg (range 35–177 kg, N = 266). Approximately 95% of patients received drug based on body weight (mg/kg), whereas the remaining patients had fixed dosing (mg). Transitioning from 0.25-mg/kg weight-based to 17.5-mg fixed dosing, exposure–safety response analysis showed that the predicted toxicity rate remains similar for patients with average body weight. However, in patients with lower/higher body weights, the range of toxicity rate was significantly tighter for the fixed dose as compared to the weight-based dose.

The model predicted the toxicity rate for hepatocellular carcinoma (HCC) patients successfully and showed lower variability across patients for fixed dose. A fixed 17.5-mg dose of linifanib was recommended for HCC patients based on the exposure-predicted safety profile.

The objective of this analysis was to identify a linifanib dose/dosing regimen that has an acceptable safety profile for a phase 3 study in HCC patients. The pharmacokinetics (PK) of linifanib was characterized from two phase 1 and three phase 2 clinical trials, evaluating linifanib as a single agent in 266 subjects from 316 enrolled patients. Covariates that have an impact on linifanib PK were identified. The derived linifanib PK parameters were used to evaluate the relationship of linifanib exposure to the safety profile, thereby selecting a dose/dosing regimen for a phase 3 study.

Studies were conducted internationally in advanced/metastatic solid tumors and leukemia patients to characterize the linifanib efficacy/safety profile. Patients received linifanib until progressive disease or intolerable toxicity across all studies (Table 3.11). A two-stage approach was utilized—first, the population PK analysis was conducted to characterize the linifanib exposure for each subject; then, linifanib C_{max} and AUC derived from the population PK were correlated with the rates of adverse events (AEs).

The data were analyzed using the NONMEM software version VI.[11] Linifanib PK was characterized by a one-compartment model with first-order absorption and first-order elimination. This model included inter-individual variability on all PK parameters and a combination of additive and proportional residual error. This model was defined as a base model and was used for the identification of covariates that influence linifanib PK. Tested covariates included body mass index (BMI), body surface area (BSA), body weight (WGT), creatinine clearance (CrCL), cancer type (HCC vs. renal cell carcinoma [RCC] vs. others), formulation (solution vs. tablet), race (Asian vs. Caucasian vs. others), and sex. Covariates were tested using an iterative forward addition ($p < 0.01$) and a backward elimination ($p < 0.001$) procedure. Using the base model as the first starting model for covariate selection, all relevant covariates were tested on apparent clearance (CL/F) and apparent volume of distribution (V/F). After completing the forward addition, the covariate that had the least significance (highest value of p, with

TABLE 3.11

Study Descriptions

Study	Phase	Study Description
M04-710	1	Open-label, multiple-dose escalation study in patients with advanced non-hematological malignancies. PK samples were collected at various time points on studies D1 and D15. Additional pre-dose samples were collected in later cycles.
M05-756	1	Multicenter, dose-escalating study in acute myelogenous leukemia and myelodysplastic syndrome patients. PK samples were collected at various time points on D1 and D8. Additional pre-dose samples were collected in later cycles.
M06-879	2	Single-arm trial in advanced HCC patients. Child-Pugh A and B patients received linifanib 0.25-mg/kg once daily and once every other day, respectively. PK samples were taken at various time points on D1 after single dose in 9 Child-Pugh A and 6 Child-Pugh B patients. Pre-dose PK samples were taken on D1 of Week 2, 4, and at the end of Week 8.
M06-880	2	NSCLC patients received oral linifanib, 0.10 or 0.25 mg/kg. Pre-dose PK samples were taken on D1 of weeks 2, 3, 4, and 5 and at the end of week 8.
M06-882	2	Patients with advanced RCC received 0.25-mg/kg QD dose. Pre-dose samples were taken on D8, D15, D29, week 8, and week 12.

D, Day; HCC, hepatocellular carcinoma; NSCLC, non–small cell lung carcinoma; PK, pharmacokinetics; RCC, renal cell carcinoma.

$p > 0.001$) was excluded in an iterative process in the backward elimination. The final model was defined as the model containing only the most significant covariate relations. Likelihood ratio test was used to compare nested models ($p < 0.01$). Goodness of fit plots were used to assess the adequacy of the final model. Robustness of the parameter estimates from the final model was also assessed using bootstrap validation.

3.4.3 Results and Conclusion

Data from patients enrolled in two phase 1 (solid tumors and acute myeloid leukemia) and three phase 2 monotherapy studies (non–small cell lung carcinoma [NSCLC], HCC, and RCC) who had PK information were used. Adverse events were graded by National Cancer Institute (NCI) Common Terminology Criteria for Adverse Events (CTCAE) V3.0.[12] Prior to the exposure–response analysis, eight common (>10%) AEs were identified as response variables—hypertension, asthenia (including fatigue), gastrointestinal–oral (mouth ulceration, odynophagia, oral pain, and paresthesia oral), gastrointestinal–abdominal disorder (abdominal discomfort, abdominal pain, abdominal pain lower, abdominal pain upper, and abdominal tenderness), diarrhea, skin toxicity 1 (dermatitis, dry skin, erythema, rash, rash follicular, rash generalized, skin disorder, skin lesion, and skin reaction), skin toxicity 2 (blisters, palmar erythema, palmar–plantar erythrodysesthesia), and proteinuria. The exposure variables (predictor) were the steady-state maximum observed concentration (C_{max}) and AUC derived from the population PK analyses. PK parameters (CL/F, V/F, and absorption rate constant [Ka]) obtained from the population PK analysis were used to simulate PK profiles for different doses or regimen at steady state assuming no dose reductions/interruptions. These PK profiles were then used to calculate the values of C_{max} and AUC at steady state. Since AEs occurring long after study drug administration were not necessarily deemed to be clinically relevant to the study drug, only data with the highest AE grade level developed within the first 8 weeks of study for each patient were included in the statistical analyses. To increase the power of statistical analyses, the AE severity grade levels as defined by the NCI-CTACE V3.0 criteria were categorized into two groups. The group was called an EVENT if the AE grade was two or higher and a NON-EVENT otherwise. A logistic regression analysis was performed for the exposure–safety response analysis for each AE.

To explore the possibility of transition from weight-based dose to fixed dose, an analysis was performed to compare the predicted AE rate after weight-based and fixed dosing. Since sex was significantly correlated to exposure (C_{max} and AUC), the analysis was done separately for male and female patients. Specifically, for each of the AEs identified (hypertension, diarrhea, proteinuria, and asthenia), predictions were computed for male and female patients separately, with heavy (110 kg), average (70 kg), and light (30 kg) body weights, respectively, for both weight-based and fixed dosing.

Since analyses based on C_{max} and AUC resulted in very similar predictions for hypertension, diarrhea, and proteinuria, the predicted event rates based on C_{max} were depicted. For asthenia, however, only AUC but not C_{max} was identified as a significant predictor for the likelihood of the event and thus the predicted event rate from AUC was used.

Of the 316 patients enrolled across five multicenter studies (cancer types: HCC 14.6%, RCC 17.1%, NSCLC 46.5%, others including breast, colon, bladder, pancreatic, head/neck, and miscellaneous, 21.8%), 266 patients with both exposure and AE data were included in the exposure–response analysis (Table 3.12). In this combined data set, 46% patients were Asian, 48% Caucasian, and 6% from other races; median body weight was 68 kg (range: 35–177 kg). Most patients were male (64%) but the population contained a significant number of female patients ($N = 83$). Additional demographic covariates considered in the population PK model were BMI (median = 24.7 kg/m^2 with range of 13.7–52.9 kg/m^2), BSA (median = 1.8 m^2 with range of 1.2–2.8 m^2), and CrCL (median = 82.4 mL/min with range of 35.3–290.3 mL/min). Most patients (87.6%) received an oral solution of linifanib, while 12.4% received a tablet formulation. Approximately 95% of patients received drug based on body weight (mg/kg), whereas the remaining patients had fixed dosing (mg).

The objective of this analysis is the correlation between linifanib exposures and safety responses. A brief description of the population PK is as follows. A one-compartment model with first order absorption and elimination described the data well. Utilizing forward and backward selections and via examination for the differences in the objective function, both body weight and sex were identified as the significant covariate for V/F (and therefore C_{max}), while sex was the only significant covariate for CL/F (therefore, AUC). Model adequacy was examined upon a goodness of fit analysis. One-thousand simulations were performed using the final population PK model. No apparent bias was observed in the model (Table 3.13).

Linifanib exposure was significantly associated with increased rates of hypertension ($p = 0.02$ for C_{max} and $p = 0.01$ for AUC), diarrhea ($p = 0.001$ for C_{max} and $p = 0.0012$ for AUC), proteinuria ($p = 0.001$ for C_{max} and $p = 0.002$ for AUC), and asthenia ($p = 0.03$ for AUC) events. The incidence rates of the remaining adverse events were not associated with linifanib exposure.

Drug exposures obtained from the population PK model were converted to a variety of dose levels after accounting for sex and body weight, thereby depicting the full scale of the dose–response relationship for body weight dosing from 0.10–0.25 mg/kg or for fixed dosing from 7.5–17.5 mg.

On the basis of exposure–response analysis, the predicted toxicity rates were calculated for both male and female patients for each AE. In this study, the average body weight was approximately 70 kg, with a range from 30 to 110 kg. Therefore, to characterize the variability among patients of different sizes, the predicted toxicity rates for 30, 70, and 110 kg were also estimated. Under the weight-based dosing scheme, heavier patients had a greater risk of toxicity as the exposure increased significantly. Transitioning from

TABLE 3.12

Patient Demographics

Study No.	Number of Patients (N)	Median Age, Years, (Range)	Median Body Weight, kg, (Range)	Gender		Race		
				Men n (%)	Women n (%)	Caucasian n (%)	Asian n (%)	Other n (%)
M04-710	33	56 (29–76)	56 (36–107)	16 (48)	17 (52)	0 (0)	31 (94)	2 (6)
M05-756	29	56 (24–81)	73 (46–128)	16 (55)	13 (45)	23 (74)	5 (17)	1 (4)
M06-879	38	63 (20–81)	58 (42–88)	31 (82)	7 (18)	1 (3)	37 (97)	0 (0)
M06-880	124	62 (33–85)	70 (35–177)	73 (59)	51 (41)	72 (58)	46 (37)	6 (5)
M06-882	42	60 (40–80)	84 (57–158)	35 (83)	7 (17)	34 (81)	1 (2)	7 (17)
All	266	61 (20–85)	68 (35–177)	171 (64)	95 (36)	130 (49)	120 (45)	16 (6)

TABLE 3.13

Population PK Parameter Estimates from the Final Model

Parameter (Unit)	Final Model Estimate (SEE)
Structural model parameters	
CL/F (L/hr) = Males	3.65 (0.13)
CL/F (L/hr) Females	2.81 (0.20)
V/F (L) = Males	96.8 (5.0)
V/F (L) = Females	71.5 (5.8)
Coefficient for weight	0.942 (0.171)
K_a (1/hr)	1.32 (0.09)
Inter-individual variability parameters	
Variance of IIV on CL/F	0.22
Variance of IIV on V/F	0.13
Residual error parameters	
Variance of proportional error term	0.06
Variance of additive error term	0.02

SEE: Standard Error of the Estimate; CL/F: apparent clearance; V/F: apparent volume of distribution; Ka: absorption rate constant.

0.25-mg/kg weight-based to 17.5-mg fixed dosing, the exposure–safety response analysis showed that the predicted hypertension rate remained similar for patients with average body weight (39% for men and 44% for women). However, in patients with lower and higher body weights, the hypertension rate range was tighter for the fixed dose (37%–42% for males and 42%–55% for females) as compared to the weight-based dose (30%–46% for males and 34%–55% for females). Similar trends were observed for diarrhea, proteinuria, and asthenia (Figure 3.5). As the likelihood of the other safety events did not appear to be associated with a change in linifanib exposure, body weight–based and fixed dosing regimens are expected to result in comparable toxicity rates for those AEs.

A one-compartment model with first order absorption and elimination described the data well. CrCl was not a significant covariate on CL/F or V/F in the final model, suggesting that patients with renal impairment do not require a different dose. A population PK analysis of the available data showed no association between hepatic function and CL/F or V/F suggesting no dose adjustment for liver-impaired patients. However, in the final model, sex was a covariate on CL/F and on V/F, indicating that males and females will have different plasma exposures for the same dose. The analysis showed that, as expected, linifanib exposure was significantly associated with toxicities manifested by anti-VEGF activities, and most noticeably, the event of hypertension. On the basis of the exposure–response model, more than 30% of patients who received 0.25-mg/kg or 17.5-mg linifanib would experience at least one event of hypertension at Grade 2 or above, which

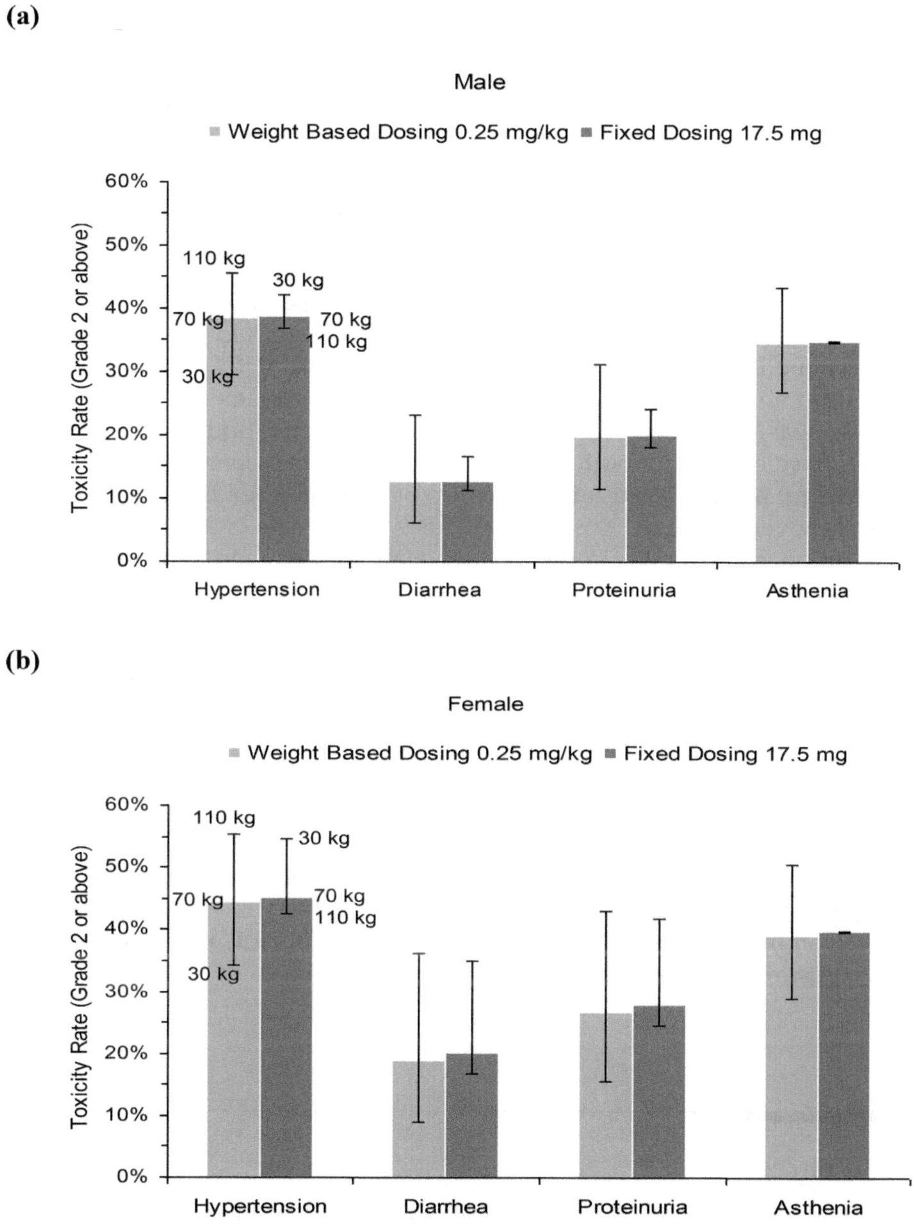

FIGURE 3.5
Comparison of predicted rates of toxicities based on C_{max} and AUC between weight-based and fixed dosing for male (a) and female (b) patients.

could require medical intervention. Indeed, the actual percentage of patients who experienced the event was 37% for all patients combined, and 34% for HCC patients. Since the exposure is associated with the toxicity rate, the risk increased for heavier patients under weight-based dosing.

Although approximately 95% of patients received drug based on body weight (mg/kg) in the linifanib clinical trials, there was an interest in administering a fixed dose instead of a body weight dose. As body weight was not a significant covariate for the CL/F and, therefore, AUC in the population PK analysis, adjusting dose by body weight would not be likely to gain additional benefit for stabilizing the overall average exposure. After the administration of a fixed dose, different C_{max} values are expected for patients with different body weights. Since the exposure (C_{max} and AUC) was significantly correlated with sex in the population PK analysis, assessment of safety (rates of AEs) was conducted for the two dosing regimens (body weight dosing versus fixed dosing) for both male and female patients separately. For all AEs considered, the predicted rates appear to be similar when linifanib is dosed by weight versus a fixed dose for patients with average body weight (70 kg). In addition, the AE rates in male patients are tighter over the weight range (30–110 kg) for fixed versus weight-based dosing. The predicted AE range for female patients was slightly higher as compared to male patients, but the AE range is still tighter over the weight range for fixed dosing regardless of the sex as compared to the weight-based dosing. These results suggest that a fixed dose would be more beneficial than a weight-based dose for the population.

In conclusion, this analysis showed that linifanib PK can be well described by a one-compartment model with first-order absorption and elimination. HCC patients had similar exposures to patients with other tumor types. Despite a vast majority of patients having received drug based on body weight (mg/kg) in phase 1 and 2, a fixed 17.5-mg starting dose of linifanib was recommended for phase 3 and is being tested in HCC patients based on the exposure-predicted safety profile.

References

1. Williams J. R. The Declaration of Helsinki and Public Health. *Bulletin of the World Health Organization* 86: 650–651, 2008.
2. QT interval LITFL ECG Library Basics, (lifeinthefastlane.com › ECG Library › ECG Basics).
3. Fridericia L. S. The Duration of Systole in the Electrocardiogram of Normal Subjects and of Patients with Heart Disease. *Acta Medica Scandinavica* 53: 469–486, 1920.

4. Food and Drug Administration. *Guidance for Industry: E14 Clinical Evaluation of QT/QTc Interval Prolongation and Proarrhythmic Potential for Non-Antiarrhythmic Drugs*. U.S. Dept. of Health and Human Services, Food and Drug Administration, Center for Drug Evaluation and Research : Center for Biologics Evaluation and Research: Rockville, MD, October 2005.
5. Chow, S. and Liu J. *Design and Analysis of Bioavailability and Bioequivalence Studies*. Marcel Dekker, 1992.
6. Gould, L. A. Group Sequential Extensions of a Standard Bioequivalence Testing Procedure. *Journal of Pharmacokinetics and Biopharmaceutics* 23(1), 1995.
7. O'Quigley J., Pepe M., and Fisher L. Continual Reassessment Method: A Practical Design for Phase 1 Clinical Trials in Cancer. *Biometrics* 46: 33–48, 1990.
8. Muler J. H., McGinn C. J., Normolle D., Lawrence T., Brown D., Hekna G., and Zalupski M. M. Phase I Trial Using a Time to Event Continual Reassessment Strategy for Dose Escalation of Cisplatin Combined with Gemcitabine and Radiation Therapy in Pancreatic Cancer. *Journal of Clinical Oncology* 22(2): 238–243, 2004.
9. Cheung Y. K. and Chappell R. Sequential Designs for Phase I Clinical Trials with Late-Onset Toxicities. *Biometrics* 56: 1177–1182, 2000.
10. Liu S. and Ning J. A Bayesian Dose-finding Design for Drug Combination Trials with Delayed Toxicities. *Bayesian Analysis* 8(3): 703–722, 2013.
11. Beal S. L., Sheiner L. B., and Boeckmann A. J. (eds) (1989–2006) *NONMEM Users Guide* (1989–2008). Icon Development Solutions: Ellicott City, MD.
12. NCI. Common Terminology Criteria for Adverse Events v3.0 (CTCAE). 2006. https://ctep.cancer.gov/protocolDevelopment/electronic_applications/docs/ctcaev3.pdf.

4

Statistical Measures of Interaction for Evaluating a Predictive Biomarker

Jaya Satgopan
Memorial Sloan Kettering Cancer Center

CONTENTS

4.1 Introduction

Our knowledge of tumor biology and preventive interventions have increased considerably in the past decade [4,17,19,30,33,36]. Nonetheless, curative therapy continues to remain elusive. Most treatments that have been developed in unselected patients offer only limited clinical benefits [7]. For example, adding bevacizumab, an antibody against *VEGF-A*, to first-line chemotherapy provides an overall survival advantage of only 1.4 months in metastatic colorectal cancer patients (median overall survival of 21.3 in the bevacizumab group and 19.9 months in the control group; [24]); adding panitumumab, an antibody against *EGFR*, to bevacizumab and chemotherapy worsens the overall survival for these patients (median overall survival of 19.4 months in the panitumumab group and 24.5 in the control group; [10]). Clearly, there is an urgent need to improve the success rates of anticancer therapies.

Recent studies have noted that certain treatments are beneficial only for individuals with specific genetic characteristics. For example, panitumumab and cetuximab monotherapies improve progression-free survival (PFS) only in *EGFR*-positive metastatic colorectal cancer patients having no *KRAS* mutation in codons 12 and 13 [2,12]. Hence, the *Table of Pharmacogenomic Biomarkers for Drug Labeling* of the Food and Drug Administration (FDA) lists *KRAS* as a treatment of these indications [16]. The term refers to any measurable indicator of biological processes; inherited and acquired mutations are types of biomarkers. The term "predictive biomarker" refers to a biomarker that can help to define populations of patients who are more likely to experience a favorable effect than similar patients without the biomarker [8].

Examples of other predictive biomarkers include *HER2* positivity for trastuzumab treatment in breast cancer, *BCR-ABL* gene translocation for imatinib treatment in chronic myeloid leukemia, and *BRAF V600E* mutation for vemurafenib treatment in melanoma [30]. Predictive biomarkers carry significant potential for defining patient populations that are likely to benefit from specific anticancer therapies. Hence, they are gaining increasing acceptance in cancer treatment [14]. However, identifying reliable predictive biomarkers for cancer remains difficult [5], and only a small number of cancer biomarkers per year have been approved for use by the FDA and the European Medical Agency [32].

One of the reasons for these difficulties is the lack of a uniform statistical standard for measuring whether a biomarker is predictive. For example, some studies have made visual use of estimates to obtain insights into whether a biomarker may be predictive, without using any quantitative measure [15]. While visual investigations are useful exploratory tools, they do not constitute a robust approach for identifying predictive biomarkers. Other studies have used the interaction between a biomarker and treatment as a measure of a predictive biomarker [2]. Indeed, recent statistical works advocate evaluating the interaction between a biomarker and treatment for identifying a predictive biomarker [3,18,20,23]. However, sometimes, interaction terms can occur in statistical models because of which the outcome is measured [29,27,34,35]. For example, traits are typically analyzed by modeling disease risk on the scale. When the true underlying risk increases as an additive function of biomarkers and exposure factors at a faster (or slower) rate than that postulated by the logistic distribution, interaction terms will be required to obtain a good fit if we model the data using the logistic link function [29,27].

In recent works, we investigated the role of interaction terms in a statistical model to identify a predictive biomarker for binary and outcomes

[11,25,26]. Our investigations showed that: (i) a biomarker can be predictive of the treatment effect even in the absence of an interaction with treatment in a logistic regression model for binary traits or a regression model for time-to-event outcomes; (ii) a biomarker is not a predictive biomarker only if the biomarker or the treatment has no effect whatsoever on the outcome; and (iii) a pragmatic approach for identifying a practically useful predictive biomarker is to evaluate how risk reduction or survival gains associated with treatment differs according to the value of the biomarker.

In this chapter we provide an overview of these results and illustrate these concepts using published data from two studies: (i) that of multiple and single primary melanomas, where the outcome is binary; and (ii) phase III of metastatic melanoma, where the outcome is time to event.

4.2 Methods

We first provide a general overview of the concept of statistical interaction between a biomarker and treatment and describe the methods separately for binary and continuous outcomes in subsequent sections.

Consider an outcome *Y*, treatment *T*, and biomarker *B* measured on every individual in a study. For ease of exposition, we consider binary *T* and *B* throughout. Additional covariates or risk factors or confounding measures such as age, sex, race, ethnicity, and other genetic and exposure factors may also be measured in each person as part of the study. The general form of a model relating *Y* to *T*, *B*, and additional covariates is given by:

$$f(Y \mid B,T) = \mu + B\beta + T\delta + BT\gamma + \text{other factors,} \tag{4.1}$$

where $f(Y \mid B,T)$ is a user-specified function of the outcome, conditional upon the risk factors, taking finite values; μ is the intercept; β and δ are the additive effects of the biomarker and the treatment, respectively, and are commonly referred to as the main effects; and γ is the nonadditive effect, also referred to as the interaction effect. The right-hand side of the model may also contain the effects of other risk factors. We consider specific forms of $f(.)$ for binary and time-to-event outcomes in later sections.

Denote $g(Y \mid B,T)$ as a function of the outcome *Y*, conditional upon *B* and *T*, taking finite values. From the fundamental theory of analysis of variance [31], the statistical interaction between a biomarker and the treatment, denoted $w(Y)$ and evaluated on the scale $g(.)$ of the outcome, takes the following general form:

$$w(Y)=\{g(Y\mid B=1,T=1)-g(Y\mid B=1,T=0)\}$$
$$-\{g(Y\mid B=0,T=1)-g(Y\mid B=0,T=0)\}. \quad (4.2)$$

The term within the first curly parentheses on the right-hand side is a contrast denoting the treatment effect among carriers of the biomarker B (i.e., $B = 1$), measured on the scale $g(.)$ of the outcome. It is the magnitude of reduction in $g(.)$ associated with treatment among individuals carrying the biomarker. The term within the second curly parentheses denotes treatment effect among noncarriers (i.e., $B = 0$). The interaction effect $w(Y)$ is the difference in the treatment effect between carriers and noncarriers. If the treatment effect is the same in carriers and noncarriers, $w(Y)$ will be equal to 0.

To determine whether B is a predictive biomarker in relation to treatment T and outcome Y, we can test the null hypothesis $H_0: w(Y)=0$ against $H_A: w(Y)\neq 0$. Rejecting H_0 in favor of H_A can be taken as an evidence that B is a predictive biomarker on the scale $g(.)$ of the outcome. Given the data from multiple individuals, we can obtain the $\hat{w}(Y)$ of $w(Y)$ by maximizing the likelihood function based on Equation (4.1) and obtain the variance $\mathrm{Var}(\hat{w}(Y))$. We can then resort to the asymptotic standard normality under the test statistic $Z(Y)=\frac{\hat{w}(Y)}{\sqrt{\mathrm{Var}(\hat{w}(Y))}}$ to test H_0 against H_A and derive a p-value.

Different choices of $g(.)$ lead to interaction effects under different scales of the outcome. For example, suppose we choose $g(.)=f(.)$, that is, evaluate interaction on the same scale under which the outcome is modeled. Then, it is evident that $w(Y)=\gamma$, that is, the interaction effect in Equation (4.2) is the same as the nonadditive term in Equation (4.1). Therefore, deciding whether B is a predictive biomarker by testing $H_0: \gamma=0$ against $H_A: \gamma\neq 0$ in Equation (4.1) makes the implicit assumption that interaction effect is defined on the scale $f(.)$ of the outcome.

In practice, it may be convenient to fit a model on the scale $f(.)$. However, it may be pragmatic to evaluate the interaction contrast $w(Y)$ under a practically meaningful scale $g(.)$ that is different from $f(.)$ to identify a predictive biomarker. A lack of statistically significant interaction under the scale $f(.)$ need not imply that $w(Y)=0$ under the scale $g(.)$. This concept has been examined for binary and time-to-event outcomes in the following sections.

4.3 Binary Outcomes

Consider a binary outcome Y. We postulate a binomial distribution for Y and assume that the risk—or the probability that Y is equal to 1—depends upon B, T, and other risk factors. A conventional approach for modeling this dependence is via logistic regression [1]. Denoting $\pi_{\text{BT}} = P(Y=1|B,T)$ as the disease conditional upon treatment and biomarker, we set $f(.)$ in the left-hand side of Equation (4.1) to be the logistic link function, given by:

$$f(Y|B,T) = \log\left\{\frac{\pi_{\text{BT}}}{1-\pi_{\text{BT}}}\right\}. \tag{4.3}$$

Analytic machinery for fitting a logistic regression model to obtain maximum likelihood estimates of the model parameters and to conduct hypothesis tests on these parameters is well-established and is implemented in most statistical software packages.

To evaluate a predictive biomarker via an interaction between a biomarker and treatment, suppose we set $g(.)$ as the logistic link function in Equation (4.2). Then, the interaction contrast $w(Y)$ is the logarithm of relative risk for disease associated with treatment according to the biomarker status and is equal to γ. Deciding whether B is a predictive biomarker by testing $H_0 : \gamma = 0$ against $H_A : \gamma \neq 0$ is equivalent to evaluating interaction contrast under the logistic scale of risk.

The parameter γ is a relative quantity in the sense that it measures disease risk relative to the baseline risk. Although this is a useful quantity, relative measures are not easy to convey to an individual patient. From the public health and patient communication perspectives, it is more appealing to assess treatment effects and their variation according to biomarker values directly on the scale of risk. Therefore, it will be pragmatic to define $g(.)$ in terms of risk by setting $g(Y|B,T) = \pi_{\text{BT}}$. Hence, the interaction contrast is given by:

$$\begin{aligned} w(Y) &= \pi_{11} - \pi_{10} - \pi_{01} + \pi_{00} \\ &= \pi_{00}\left\{\frac{\pi_{11}}{\pi_{00}} - \frac{\pi_{10}}{\pi_{00}} - \frac{\pi_{10}}{\pi_{00}} + 1\right\}. \end{aligned} \tag{4.4}$$

Here π_{00} can be interpreted as the baseline risk, that is, risk among untreated noncarriers. For a rare disease, we may approximate the relative risk terms π_{jk}/π_{00}, $j,k \in \{0,1\}$, in terms of odds ratios. Hence, it follows from Equations (4.1) and (4.3) that:

$$w(Y) = \pi_{00} \times \{\exp(\beta+\delta+\gamma) - \exp(\beta) - \exp(\delta) + 1\}. \tag{4.5}$$

In the epidemiology literature, the quantity $\exp(\beta+\delta+\gamma) - \exp(\beta) - \exp(\delta) + 1$ is referred to as the "Relative Excess Risk due to Interaction" and abbreviated as RERI [21,37]. Assuming that the baseline risk π_{00} is nonzero, testing $H_0: w(Y)=0$ against $H_A: w(Y)\neq 0$ on the risk scale is equivalent to testing $H_0: \text{RERI}=0$ against $H_A: \text{RERI}\neq 0$. We can estimate RERI using the maximum likelihood estimates β, δ, and γ from a logistic regression model, obtain the variance estimate using the Delta method, test the null hypothesis $H_0: \text{RERI}=0$ against $H_A: \text{RERI}\neq 0$, and obtain the p-value to determine the statistical significance of RERI or, equivalently, $w(Y)$ on the scale of risk [37].

Note that RERI need not be equal to 0 even when $\gamma=0$, that is, we can have a nonzero interaction effect on the scale of risk even when the interaction effect is 0 on the logistic scale [9,22]. When $\gamma=0$, RERI = 0 only when $\beta=0$ or $\delta=0$ [26]. Note that when $\gamma=0$, RERI = 0 implies that $\{\exp(\beta)-1\}\{\exp(\delta)-1\}=0$. This equation holds only when $\beta=0$ or $\delta=0$. Conversely, when $\gamma=0$ and, say, $\beta=0$, it immediately follows that RERI = 0.

Taken together, these observations show that the absence of an interaction effect in a logistic regression model does not automatically imply a lack of interaction on another scale of the outcome—particularly, on the risk scale. Therefore, we can have a predictive biomarker on the risk scale of the outcome even in the absence of an interaction effect on the logistic scale.

Note that testing the null hypothesis of no interaction on the logistic scale involves testing a single parameter γ. In contrast, RERI depends upon three parameters: β, δ, and γ. Hence, the variance of RERI will be affected by the variability in β and δ in addition to that of γ. This could affect the power to test an interaction effect based on RERI. Therefore, instead of relying on a hypothesis test to detect a predictive biomarker, we may estimate $P(\gamma>0)$ and $P(\text{RERI}>0)$ and suppose that there is noteworthy evidence for a predictive biomarker on the logistic and risk scales, respectively, when these probabilities exceed some user-specified threshold—for example, when these probabilities exceed 90%. Since γ and RERI may also take negative values, we suggest estimating the maximum probabilities $\max\{P(\gamma>0),P(\gamma<0)\}$ and $\max\{P(\text{RERI}>0),P(\text{RERI}<0)\}$. Since estimating these probabilities is not straightforward, we suggest using the following procedure. Given the data on n cases and controls, sample n individuals with replacement and estimate γ and RERI for this sampled data set. Repeat this sampling procedure B times (for example, B = 1,000) and estimate $P(\gamma>0)$ and $P(\text{RERI}>0)$ as the proportions of γs and RERIs, respectively, from the sampled data that are greater than 0. Estimate $P(\gamma<0)$ and $P(\text{RERI}<0)$ in a similar manner, and obtain the maximum probabilities. This concept is based on a recent work, where we used such maximum probabilities to measure the strength of association between putative risk factors and disease outcome [28].

These concepts are illustrated in the next section using published data from a case–control study of melanoma.

4.3.1 Illustrative Example—A Case–Control Study of Melanoma

Kricker et al. [13] reported a case–control study of melanoma with individuals having single primary melanoma as controls and those with multiple primary melanomas as cases. We illustrate the concepts described earlier using sun exposure and the *MC1R* gene measured in 743 cases and 1,525 controls. Sun exposure of each person is binary, indicating the presence or absence of at least 814 kJ/m^2 of early-life ambient ultraviolet averaged at birth and age 10 (see Kricker et al. [13] for details). The binary biomarker of each person is the presence or absence of at least one red hair color variant in the *MC1R* gene. We use these data to examine whether *MC1R* may be a predictive biomarker for sun exposure in melanoma, that is, whether the effect of sun exposure on melanoma varies according to the level of *MC1R*.

Kricker et al. [13] examined the association between risk for second primary melanoma, *MC1R*, and sun exposure by adjusting for several factors such as age and sex. However, since the full data set from their study is not readily available from their paper, we illustrate the concepts described earlier using the published data reported in Table 3 of Kricker et al. [13], which is reproduced in Table 4.1.

The additive effects of *MC1R*, sun exposure, and their interaction effect on the logistic scale, denoted by β, δ, and γ, respectively, can be obtained by fitting a logistic regression model to these data. The maximum likelihood estimate of γ is 0.14 (standard error = 0.18), which is not significantly different from 0 at the 5% level (p-value = 0.44). Thus, there is no significant evidence that *MC1R* is a predictive biomarker for sun exposure on the logistic scale. The maximum likelihood estimate of RERI is 0.55 (standard error = 0.29), which is not significantly different from 0 at the 5% level (p-value = 0.06).

Figure 4.1 shows a histogram of 1,000 bootstrap estimates of γ and RERI. On the basis of these bootstrap estimates, we have $P(\gamma > 0) = 0.79 = 1 - P(\gamma < 0)$ and $P(\text{RERI} > 0) = 0.98 = 1 - P(\text{RERI} < 0)$. Hence, the maximum probabilities corresponding to γ and RERI are 0.79 and 0.98, respectively. Using a threshold of 90% probability, these estimates suggest noteworthy evidence for an interaction on the scale of risk, but not on the logistic scale.

TABLE 4.1

Data from a Case–Control Study of Melanoma Published in Table 3 of Kricker et al.

MC1R	Sun Exposure	Controls	Cases
No R	No	468	148
	Yes	330	166
Yes R	No	415	181
	Yes	312	248

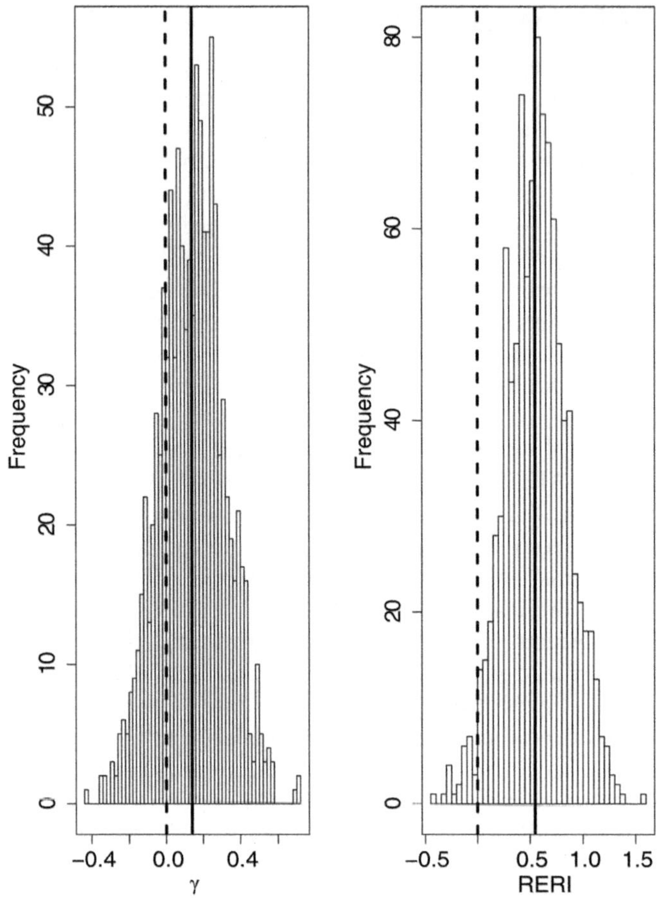

FIGURE 4.1
Bootstrap estimates of γ (left panel) and RERI (right panel) for the melanoma case–control data. The bold vertical lines show the maximum likelihood estimates 0.14 for γ and 0.55 for RERI from the observed data. The dashed vertical lines show the null γ and RERI values of 0.

Computer commands in the R programming language for obtaining these results are given in Section 0.1.

4.4 Time-To-Event Outcomes

Consider a time-to-event outcome Y, which is the observed time at which the endpoint occurs in a person or if the person does not have the endpoint, their last follow-up time. As before, let B and T denote binary biomarker and treatment or exposure, respectively.

Denote $S(Y \mid B,T)$ as the survival probability, that is, the probability that a person survives beyond time Y, given B and T. We can estimate this probability using the Kaplan–Meier approach [6], which is implemented in most statistical software packages.

Let $\lambda(Y \mid B,T)$ denote the hazard of event at time Y, given B and T. From the fundamental concepts of survival analysis [6], we have: $S(Y \mid B,T) = \exp\left\{-\int_0^Y \lambda(u \mid B,T)\,du\right\}$. A common approach for modeling disease hazard as a function of B and T is the proportional hazards regression model given by:

$$\log\{\lambda(Y \mid B,T)\} = \log\{\lambda_0(Y)\} + B\beta + T\delta + BT\gamma, \tag{4.6}$$

where $\lambda_0(Y)$ denotes the baseline hazard at time Y. In the notation of Equation (4.1), we have $f(Y \mid B,T) = \log\{\lambda(Y \mid B,T)\}$ and $\mu = \log\{\lambda_0(Y)\}$. Analytic machinery for fitting this model to estimate β, δ, γ, and software packages for fitting the proportional hazards model are widely available.

To evaluate a predictive biomarker, we consider two scales of outcome to define the interaction effect $w(Y)$. First, we measure the interaction effect on the logarithm of the hazard scale by defining $g(Y \mid B,T) = \log\{\lambda(Y \mid B,T)\}$ in Equation (4.2). Thus, the interaction effect is the logarithm of hazard ratios. When the true disease hazard follows a proportional hazards model given by Equation (4.6), we have $w(Y) = \gamma$, which does not depend upon Y. Testing whether B is a predictive biomarker on the logarithm of hazard scale is equivalent to testing the null hypothesis $H_0 : \gamma = 0$ against the alternative $H_A : \gamma \neq 0$, which can be done using statistical software packages that implement proportional hazards regression model. When $\gamma = 0$, B is not a predictive biomarker on the logarithm of hazard scale.

In practice, however, the effect of treatment and variation in treatment effect can depend upon time. For example, the effect of a treatment may be best realized only after a certain time. From this viewpoint, evaluating a predictive biomarker on the hazard scale using a proportional hazards framework may not be a clinically useful approach. Further, the hazard function is not easily interpretable during a dialog between a clinical practitioner and a patient. The probability of surviving beyond a particular time point based on biomarker values and treatment assignment is an attractive measure that can be more easily communicated to a patient than the hazard ratio. Hence, we define the interaction effect $w(Y)$ on the survival probability scale by defining $g(Y \mid B,T) = S(Y \mid B,T)$.

On the survival probability scale, the treatment effect for a given B measures the increase in survival probability associated with treatment in that biomarker group. The interaction measures the difference in survival gains between the carrier and noncarrier biomarker groups, which is analogous to RERI. Unlike the interaction effect defined on the logarithm of hazard scale and under the proportional hazards framework, the interaction effect on the survival probability scale depends upon the time point Y. The survival probabilities and, hence, $w(Y)$ can be estimated using the Kaplan–Meier approach for a given Y, although, in principle, they may also be estimated via a proportional hazards regression model. In this chapter, we use the Kaplan–Meier approach to estimate the survival probabilities at the desired time Y, where Y may be chosen according to clinical relevance such as six-month or one-year survival probabilities or using summary such as the median survival time based on the full data set.

Note that, under the proportional hazards framework, the interaction effect on the survival probability scale can be written as [25]:

$$w(Y)=\{A_0(Y)\}^{\exp(\beta+\delta+\gamma)}-\{A_0(Y)\}^{\exp(\beta)}-\{A_0(Y)\}^{\exp(\delta)}+\{A_0(Y)\}, \quad (4.7)$$

where $\{A_0(Y)\}=\exp\left\{-\int_0^Y \lambda_0(u)du\right\}$. When $\gamma=0$, the right-hand side is equal to 0 only when β or δ is equal to 0. This suggests that, when there is no interaction in a proportional hazards model, we can have a nonzero interaction effect on the survival probability scale. Therefore, we can have a predictive biomarker on the survival probability scale even when there is no interaction effect on the logarithm of hazard scale.

Once the survival difference is estimated using the Kaplan–Meier approach, we can evaluate whether B is a predictive biomarker by testing H_0 : survival difference $= 0$ against the alternative H_A : survival difference $\neq 0$ via a normal approximation to the test statistic, as noted earlier.

Even though we estimate the survival difference using the Kaplan–Meier estimates of survival probabilities, it can be noted from the proportional hazards formulation given in Equation (4.7) that the interaction effect on the survival probability scale can depend upon both additive and nonadditive parameters. This could potentially affect the power to detect an interaction effect on the survival probability scale. Therefore, as before, we suggest a bootstrap approach to investigate noteworthy evidence for the presence of a predictive biomarker as an alternative to hypothesis testing on the logarithm of hazards and survival probability scales. As in the case of binary outcomes, this approach involves estimating the interaction effects on the logarithm of hazard and survival probability scales by repeatedly sampling with replacement from the observed data to estimate the corresponding maximum probabilities.

These concepts are illustrated in the next section using digitized data from a published clinical trial of metastatic melanoma.

4.4.1 Illustrative Example—A Phase III Trial of Metastatic Melanoma

Nivolumab (abbreviated N), a programmed death 1 (PD-1) checkpoint inhibitor, and ipilimumab (abbreviated I), a cytotoxic T-lymphocyte-associated antigen 4 (CTLA-4) checkpoint inhibitor are used in the treatment of metastatic melanoma. Recently, Larkin et al. [15] reported the results of a double-blinded phase III clinical trial of metastatic melanoma patients, where 945 patients were randomized in a 1:1:1 ratio to N monotherapy, C monotherapy, and N + I combination therapy. Randomization was stratified according to the binary (positive or negative) status of programmed death 1 ligand (PD-L1) expression, which could be evaluated for 843 patients. The main objective of this study was to assess the effect of treatment on PFS, measured as months since treatment assignment. To illustrate the methods described, we use data from 565 patients randomized to N or I monotherapies, their PD-L1 status, and PFS.

Since the full data from this phase III trial is not available, we digitized the figures reported in Larkin et al. [15] and extracted approximate patient-level data on PFS time, PFS status, treatment group, and PD-L1–positivity status in 565 patients receiving N or I monotherapy. Details of the digital extraction process and software packages used are described elsewhere [25] and will not be repeated here. The digitized data are available upon request from the author of this chapter.

The median survival time based on 565 patients is 3.95 months. The sample sizes in the N and I treatment groups and PD-L1 status based on the digitally extracted data are given in Table 4.2. Figure 4.2 shows the Kaplan–Meier estimates of PFS for PD-L1–positive (n = 155) and PD-L1–negative (n = 410) patients. It is evident that patients receiving N have better PFS than those receiving I, regardless of the PD-L1 status. On the basis of a proportional hazards model, the maximum likelihood estimate of the effect of I monotherapy (baseline is N monotherapy) on the logarithm of hazard scale is 0.53 in the PD-L1–negative group and 0.89 in the PD-L1–positive group. Thus, the magnitude of treatment effect on the logarithm of hazard scale is higher for the PD-L1–positive than the PD-L1–negative group. The effect of interaction on the logarithm of hazard scale is 0.36 (= 0.89 – 0.53; standard error = 0.25), which is not significantly different from 0 at the 5% level (p-value = 0.15).

Next, we calculate treatment and interaction effects on the survival probability scale at the median survival time of Y = 3.95 months. This choice of Y is unbiased in the sense that it uses the complete data set of

TABLE 4.2

Summary Based on Digitized Data from the Phase III Trial of Metastatic Melanoma of Larkin et al.

PD-L1	Treatment	Total Patients	Total Events
Negative	Nivolumab	208	127
	Ipilimumab	202	156
Positive	Nivolumab	80	32
	Ipilimumab	75	53

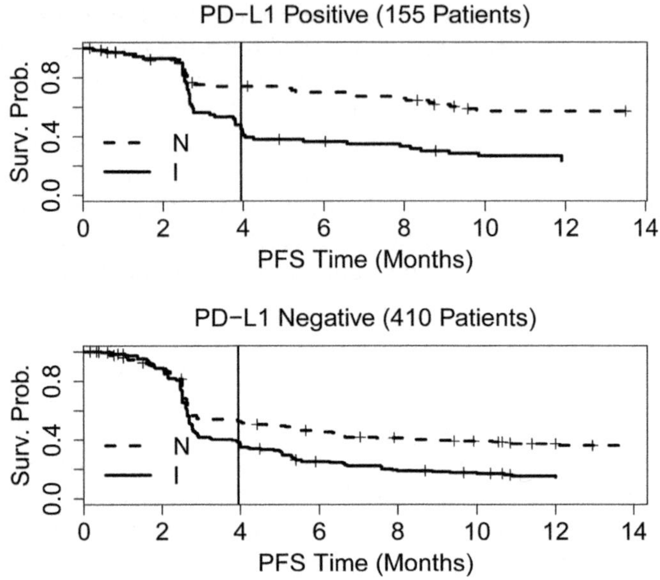

FIGURE 4.2
Kaplan–Meier estimates of PFS probabilities for PD-L1–positive (top panel) and negative (bottom panel) metastatic melanoma patients receiving nivolumab (N; dashed line) and ipilimumab (I; bold line) treatments. The median survival time of 3.95 months based on all the 565 patients is shown as a vertical line.

565 patients and does not depend on PFS time according to the PD-L1 status and treatment groups. The treatment effect on the survival probability scale is –0.29 in the PD-L1–positive group, that is, PFS at 3.95 months is reduced by 29% for PD-L1–positive patients receiving I monotherapy compared to those receiving N monotherapy. The corresponding treatment effect for PD-L1–negative patients is –0.14. The interaction effect is –0.15 (= –0.29 + 0.15; standard error = 0.092), which is not significantly different from 0 at the 5% level (p-value = 0.11). Thus, these data do not provide significant evidence that PD-L1 expression is a predictive biomarker for N versus I monotherapy in metastatic melanoma patients on the survival probability scale.

Figure 4.1 shows a histogram of 1,000 bootstrap estimates of interactions on the logarithm of hazard scale (i.e., γ) and survival probability scale (i.e., survival difference). On the basis of these bootstrap estimates, we have $P(\gamma > 0) = 0.93 = 1 - P(\gamma < 0)$ and $P(\text{survival difference} < 0) = 0.93 = 1 - P(\text{survival difference} > 0)$. On a threshold of 90% probability, these estimates suggest noteworthy evidence for an interaction on both the scales considered.

Computer commands in the R programming language to obtain these results are given in Section 0.2.

4.5 Concluding Remarks

There is considerable interest in evaluating the statistical interaction between a biomarker and the treatment for identifying a predictive biomarker. However, the presence of an interaction may depend upon the scale on which the outcome is measured. In this chapter, we have examined different scales of outcome to evaluate an interaction between a biomarker and the treatment for binary and time-to-event outcomes. Our investigations are built on extensive studies of interactions in the epidemiology literature and in our prior works [11,22,21,26,25,37].

The evaluation of the interaction between a biomarker and treatment on a practically interpretable scale is an important first step in identifying a predictive biomarker. However, the presence of such an interaction alone is not sufficient for using a biomarker to make treatment decisions. Validation of the interaction using external data is crucial. Several additional follow-up investigations are also required before a biomarker can be used to make treatment decisions in practice. These investigations include evaluating the cost–benefit aspects of using a biomarker in practice and evaluating toxicities associated with treatment, to name a few.

Our illustrative example of a case–control study of melanoma suggests that there is a noteworthy interaction between *MC1R* and sun exposure on the risk scale. From a practical standpoint, this noteworthy observation would mean that interventions such as education strategies about reducing sun exposure as a way to reduce the risk of multiple primary melanomas are broadly important for all patients; however, a more specialized education to this end may be provided to individuals carrying a red hair color variant in *MC1R*. Taken at face value, this implies that every patient must be tested for the presence of a red hair color variant in *MC1R*, and educational intervention strategies about reducing sun exposure can be tailored according to the presence or absence of this variant. Thus, there is a cost associated with genetic testing to decide the intervention strategy. In practice, however, the cost–benefit aspects of tailoring intervention strategies according to the value of a biomarker must be explored in detail before they can be implemented. Further research is required on cost–benefit aspects of predictive biomarkers and is not pursued here.

Our illustrative example of a phase III clinical trial of metastatic melanoma suggests that there is a noteworthy interaction between treatment and PD-L1 on both logistic and survival probability scales. While nivolumab treatment is associated with improved PFS relative to ipilimumab treatment in both PD-L1–positive and PD-L1–negative patients, the improvement is greater in PD-L1–positive than PD-L1–negative patients. Taken at face value, this implies that PD-L1–positive patients are likely to benefit better from nivolumab treatment than PD-L1–negative patients. Whether this implies that PD-L1–positive patients alone may be treated with nivolumab is an important question, but one that requires a deeper understanding of the data and the results. In our example, nivolumab improves PFS regardless of PD-L1 status (see Figure 4.3), which suggests that, despite a noteworthy interaction, nivolumab treatment may be appropriate for all patients regardless of their PD-L1 status. Further, any toxicities associated with treatment, over and above its statistical interaction with a biomarker, can also play a crucial role in deciding whether that treatment should be administered to patients regardless of or according to the biomarker status. Further research is required on aspects surrounding toxicities to evaluate a predictive biomarker and is not pursued here.

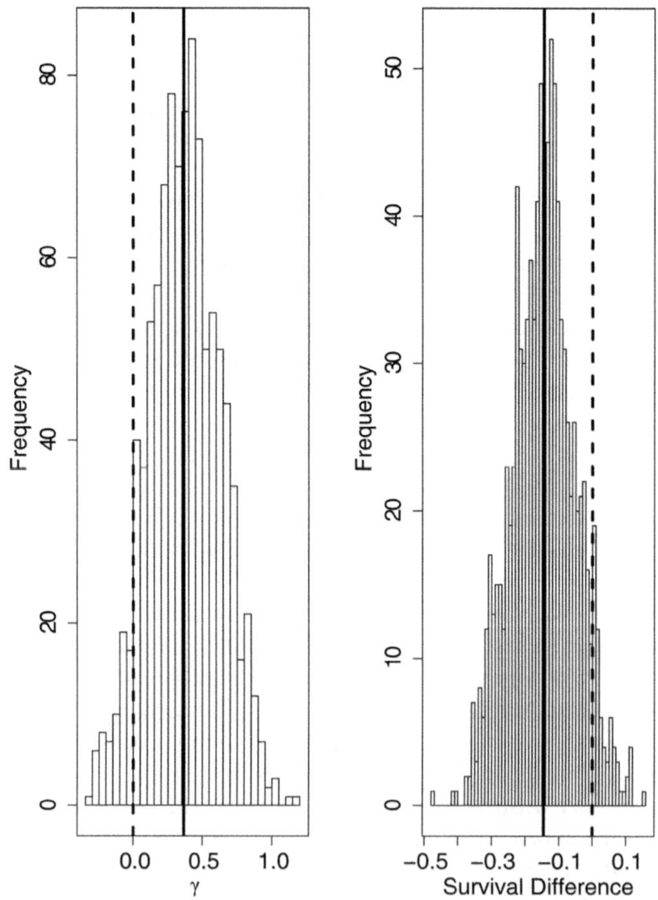

FIGURE 4.3
Bootstrap estimates of interactions based on the logarithm of hazard scale (γ; left panel) and the survival probability scale (survival difference; right panel) based on digitized data for patients receiving nivolumab and ipilimumab monotherapies in the metastatic melanoma phase III trial. The bold vertical lines show the maximum likelihood estimates 0.36 and −0.15 for interactions on the logarithm of hazard and survival scales, respectively, from the digitized data. The dashed vertical lines show the null interaction effects of 0.

The ideas in this chapter are presented in the context of a binary biomarker and a binary treatment. Advances in biotechnology allow us to measure a large number of biomarkers—for example, genome-wide evaluation of inherited and acquired mutations and gene expressions. Further research is required in the areas of statistical and computational models to assess variation in treatment effects associated with multiple biomarkers and is not addressed here. For a time-to-event endpoint, the interaction on survival probability scale is evaluated at a specific time point. The time point must not be chosen conveniently after looking at the outcome according to the biomarker and treatment groups. Further research is required on the choice of an optimal time point to evaluate a predictive biomarker and is not discussed here.

In summary, investigating an interaction between a biomarker and treatment in relation to an outcome as a strategy for identifying a predictive biomarker, while important, must proceed with care. This is because the presence of an interaction may depend upon the scale on which an outcome is measured. Several open quantitative problems remain in the area of predictive biomarkers, warranting further statistical research on this topic.

Acknowledgment

This chapter benefited from ideas developed in recent publications with colleagues from Memorial Sloan Kettering Cancer Center—particularly, Satagopan, Iasonos, and Zhou [26], Iasonos, Chapman, and Satagopan [11], and Satagopan and Iasonos [25].

Computer Programs

0.1 R Commands for Analyzing the Kricker et al. Melanoma Data with Binary Outcome

```
> n.control = c(468, 330, 415, 312)
> n.case = c(148, 166, 181, 248)
>
> y = c(rep(1, sum(n.case)), rep(0, sum(n.control)))
>
>mclr = c(rep(0, n.case[1] + n.case[2]),
          rep(1, n.case[3] + n.case[4]),
          rep(0, n.control[1] + n.control[2]),
          rep(1, n.control[3] + n.control[4]))
```

```
>
> sun.exp = c(rep(0,n.case[1]), rep(1,n.case[2]),
            rep(0,n.case[3]), rep(1,n.case[4]),
            rep(0,n.control[1]), rep(1,n.control[2]),
            rep(0,n.control[3]),rep(1,n.control[4]))
>
> full.fit = glm(y~mc1r * sun.exp, family="binomial")
>
> round(summary(full.fit)$coeff, 2)
              Estimate Std. Error z value Pr(>|z|)
(Intercept)      -1.15       0.09  -12.21     0.00
mc1r              0.32       0.13    2.48     0.01
sun.exp           0.46       0.13    3.46     0.00
mc1r:sun.exp      0.14       0.18    0.75     0.45

> beta = round(summary(full.fit)$coeff["mc1r", "Estimate"], 2)
> delta=round(summary(full.fit)$coeff["sun.exp","Estimate"], 2)
> gamma = round(summary(full.fit)$coeff["mc1r:sun.exp","Estim
ate"],                              2)
> se.gamma = round(sqrt(
              summary(full.fit)$cov.scaled["mc1r:sun.exp",
                                        "mc1r:sun.exp"]), 2)
> gamma.p.value = round(2*(1-pnorm(abs(gamma/se.gamma))), 2)
> gamma.result = c(gamma, se.gamma, gamma.p.value)
> names(gamma.result) = c("estimate",  "s.e", "p-value")
> gamma.result
estimate      s.e  p-value
    0.14     0.18     0.44

################# RERI ############
> reri = exp(beta + delta + gamma) - exp(beta) - exp(delta) + 1
> var.mat.par = summary(full.fit)$cov.scaled[-1,-1]
> deriv.vector = matrix( c(exp(beta+delta+gamma) - exp(beta),
+                          exp(beta+delta+gamma) - exp(delta),
+                          exp(beta+delta+gamma)), nrow=1)
> reri.se = sqrt(as.vector(deriv.vector %*% var.mat.par %*%
                         t(deriv.vector)))
> test.reri = reri / reri.se
> reri.p = 2 * (1-pnorm(abs(test.reri)))
> reri.result = c(reri, reri.se, reri.p)
> names(reri.result) = c("reri", "s.e", "p-value")
> round(reri.result, 2)
   reri     s.e p-value
   0.55    0.29    0.06

#############
#
# The commands to get the bootstrap estimates of
# maximum probabilities are not described in detail.
# Only a brief outline is given.
```

```
#
##############
> obs.data = data.frame(y=y, mclr=mclr, sun.exp=sun.exp)
> n.boot = 1000
> reri.boot = NULL
> gamma.boot = NULL
> for(i in 1:n.boot){
+  print(paste("i is ", i))
+  sample.id = sample(1:nrow(obs.data),nrow(obs.data),replace=T)
+   boot.data = obs.data[sample.id,]
######
#
# apply the given analyses to the data in boot.data
#
# collect gamma andreri into the vectors gamma.boot and reri.boot
#
######
+ }

> max(length(which(gamma.boot>0))/n.boot,
+     length(which(gamma.boot<0))/n.boot)
[1] 0.786
> max(length(which(reri.boot>0))/n.boot,
+     length(which(reri.boot<0))/n.boot)
[1] 0.975
```

0.2 R Commands for Analyzing the Larkin et al. Metastatic Melanoma Data with Time-To-Event Outcome

```
#############
#
# The object larkin.nivo.ipi.data contains the required data.
##############

#############
# A sample view of the first 10 rows of this data set
# is given here. Column 1 is PFS time. Column 2 is
# binary indicator for event. Column 3 is treatment
# arm number indicating the treatment and pdl1-status
# combination. Column 5 is pdfl1.status of a patient, and
# Column 6 is the patient's treatment type.
#
#############
> larkin.nivo.ipi.data[1:10,]
    time event tmt.arm.number pdl1.status treatment.type
1  0.678     1  nivo.pdl1.neg    negative      nivolumab
2  0.678     1  nivo.pdl1.neg    negative      nivolumab
3  0.678     1  nivo.pdl1.neg    negative      nivolumab
```

```
4  0.678     1  nivo.pdl1.neg    negative      nivolumab
5  0.678     1  nivo.pdl1.neg    negative      nivolumab
6  0.905     1  nivo.pdl1.neg    negative      nivolumab
7  0.910     1  nivo.pdl1.neg    negative      nivolumab
8  0.939     1  nivo.pdl1.neg    negative      nivolumab
9  1.140     1  nivo.pdl1.neg    negative      nivolumab
10 1.140     1  nivo.pdl1.neg    negative      nivolumab

######
# get median survival time
######
> full.fit = survfit(Surv(time, event)~1, data=larkin.nivo.ipi.
data)
> median.surv.time =
+   summary(full.fit)$time[which(summary(full.fit)$surv< 0.50)
[1]]
>
> median.surv.time
[1] 3.95

######
###### fit proportional hazards regression model to estimate
interaction
###### effect on the logarithm of hazard scale
######
> larkin.cox = coxph(Surv(time, event)~pdl1.status *
+                     (treatment.type=="ipilimumab"),
+                     data=larkin.nivo.ipi.data)
>
> tmt.effect.pdl1.neg = summary(larkin.cox)$coeff[2,1]
> tmt.effect.pdl1.neg
[1] 0.5269689
>
> tmt.effect.pdl1.pos = summary(larkin.cox)$coeff[2,1] +
+                                   summary(larkin.
cox)$coeff[3,1]
> tmt.effect.pdl1.pos
[1] 0.8913867
>
> interaction.log.hazard = summary(larkin.cox)$coeff[3,]
> interaction.log.hazard
     coef exp(coef)  se(coef)          z  Pr(>|z|)
0.3644177 1.4396755 0.2543037 1.4330023 0.1518572

> ########### interaction on the survival probability scale
##########
>
> fit.all = survfit(Surv(larkin.nivo.ipi.data$time,
+                               larkin.nivo.ipi.data$event) ~
+                     larkin.nivo.ipi.data$tmt.arm.number)
```

```
>
> fit.all.result = cbind(fit.all$time, fit.all$surv, fit.
all$std.err)
> stratum.size = cumsum(fit.all$strata)
> n1 = stratum.size[1]
> n2 = stratum.size[2]
> n3 = stratum.size[3]
> n4 = stratum.size[4]
>
> stratum.1 = fit.all.result[1:n1,]
> stratum.2 = fit.all.result[(n1+1):n2,]
> stratum.3 = fit.all.result[(n2+1):n3,]
> stratum.4 = fit.all.result[(n3+1):n4,]
>
> S11 = stratum.4[which(stratum.4[,1]>median.surv.time )[1]-1,]
> S10 = stratum.3[which(stratum.3[,1]>median.surv.time )[1]-1,]
> S01 = stratum.2[which(stratum.2[,1]>median.surv.time )[1]-1,]
> S00 = stratum.1[which(stratum.1[,1]>median.surv.time )[1]-1,]
>
#########
# the standard error returned by the survfit object is the
# standard error for log survival probability. the variance
# for survival probability is, therefore, (surv.prob* std.
error)^2,
# by delta method. therefore, variance of S11 - S10 - S01 + S00
# is calculated in the var.val object, as follows.
#########
> var.val = (S11[2] * S11[3])^2 + (S10[2] * S10[3])^2 +
+           (S01[2] * S01[3])^2 + (S00[2] * S00[3])^2
>
> tmt.effect.pdl1.pos = S11[2] - S10[2]
> tmt.effect.pdl1.neg = S01[2] - S00[2]
> interaction.surv.prob = tmt.effect.pdl1.pos - tmt.effect.
pdl1.neg
>
> test.stat = interaction.surv.prob / sqrt(var.val)
> test.p = 2 * (1 - pnorm(abs(test.stat)))
>
> interaction.surv.prob.scale =
+     c(interaction.surv.prob, sqrt(var.val), test.p)
> names(interaction.surv.prob.scale) =
+     c("int.effect", "std.err", "p-value")
>
> tmt.effect.pdl1.pos
[1] -0.2898321
> tmt.effect.pdl1.neg
[1] -0.1444108
> interaction.surv.prob.scale
 int.effect     std.err    p-value
-0.14542130  0.09223076  0.11486192
```

```
#############
#
# The commands to get bootstrap estimates
#  are not described in detail.
# Only a brief outline is given as follows.
#
##############
> n.boot = 1000
> surv.diff.boot = NULL
> surv.gamma.boot = NULL
> for(i in 1:n.boot){
+  print(paste("i is ", i))
+  sample.id = sample(1:nrow(larkin.nivo.ipi.data),
+                            nrow(larkin.nivo.ipi.
data), replace=T)
+   boot.data = larkin.nivo.ipi.data[sample.id,]
######
#
# apply the given analyses to the data in boot.data
#
# collect gamma and survival difference into
# vectors surv.gamma.boot and surv.diff.boot.
#
######
+ }

> max(length(which(surv.gamma.boot>0))/n.boot,
+     length(which(surv.gamma.boot<0))/n.boot)
[1] 0.932
>
> max(length(which(surv.diff.boot>0))/n.boot,
+     length(which(surv.diff.boot<0))/n.boot)
[1] 0.934
>
```

References

1. A. Agresti. *Categorical Data Analysis.* John Wiley and Sons, Hoboken, NJ, 2002.
2. R. G. Amado, M. Wolf, M. Peeters, et al. Wild-type KRAS is required for panitumumab efficacy in patients with metastatic colorectal cancer. *Journal of Clinical Oncology,* 26:1626–1634, 2008.
3. K. V. Ballman. Biomarker: predictive or prognostic. *Journal of Clinical Oncology,* 33:3968–3971, 2015.
4. D. T. Bishop, F. Demenais, M. M. Ilies, et al. Genome-wide association study identifies three loci associated with melanoma risk. *Nature Genetics,* 41:920–925, 2009.

5. M. Buyse, D. J. Sargent, A. Grothey, et al. Biomarkers and surrogate end points - the challenge of statistical validation. *Nature Reviews Clinical Oncology*, 7:309–317, 2010.
6. D. Collett. *Modeling Survival Data in Medical Research*. Chapman and Hall, NY, 2008.
7. A. De Gramont, S. Watson, L. M. Ellis, et al. Pragmatic issues in biomarker evaluation for targeted therapies in cancer. *Nature Reviews Clinical Oncology*, 12:197–212, 2015.
8. FDA-NIH Biomarker Working Group. BEST (Biomarkers, EndpointS, and other Tools) Resource. Available from http://www.ncbi.nlm.nih.gov/books/NBK326791/, 2016.
9. S. S. Han, P. S. Rosenberg, M. Garcia-Closas, et al. Likelihood ratio test for detecting gene (G) - environment (E) interactions under an additive risk model exploiting G-E independence for case-control data. *American Journal of Epidemiology*, 176:1060–1067, 2012.
10. J. R. Hecht, E. Mitchell, T. Chidiac, et al. A randomized phase IIIb trial of chemotherapy, bevacizumab, and panitumumab compared with chemotherapy and bevacizumab alone for metastatic colorectal cancer. *Journal of Clinical Oncology*, 27:672–680, 2009.
11. A. Iasonos, P. B. Chapman, and J. M. Satagopan. Quantifying treatment benefit in molecular subgroups to assess a predictive biomarker. *Clinical Cancer Research*, 22:2114–2120, 2016.
12. C. S. Karapetis, S. Khambata-Ford, S. Jonker, et al. K-ras mutations and benefit from cetuximab in advanced colorectal cancer. *New England Journal of Medicine*, 359:1757–1765, 2008.
13. A. Kricker, B. K. Armstrong, C. Goumas, et al. MC1R genotype may modify the effect of sun exposure on melanoma risk in the GEM study. *Cancer Causes and Control*, 21:2137–2147, 2010.
14. N. B. La Thangue and D. J. Kerr. Predictive biomarkers: a paradigm shift towards personalized cancer medicine. *Nature Reviews Clinical Oncology*, 8:587–596, 2011.
15. J. Larkin, V. Chiarion-Sileni, R. Gonzalez, et al. Combined nivolumab and ipilimumab or monotherapy in untreated melanoma. *New England Journal of Medicine*, 373:23–34, 2015.
16. C. Lee Ventola. Role of pharmacogenomic biomarkers in predicting and improving drug response. *Pharmacy and Therapeutics*, 38:545–560, 2013. Table accessed on July 28, 2016 from https://www.fda.gov/%20Drugs/ScienceResearch/ucm572698.
17. R. J. MacInnis, M. C. Pike, and J. L. Hopper. Risk-reducing surgery in hereditary breast and ovarian cancer. *New England Journal of Medicine*, 374:2403–2404, 2016.
18. H. M. Mackey and T. Bengtsson. Sample size and threshold estimation for clinical trials with predictive biomarkers. *Contemporary Clinical Trials*, 36:664–672, 2013.
19. M. C. Pike, C. L. Pearce, and A. H. Wu. Prevention of cancers of the breast, endometrium and ovary. *Oncogene*, 23:6379–6391, 2004.
20. M. C. Polley, B. Freidlin, E. L. Korn, et al. Statistical and practical considerations for clinical evaluation of predictive biomarkers. *Journal of the National Cancer Institute*, 105:1677–1683, 2013.
21. K. J. Rothman, S. Greenland, and T. L. Lash. *Modern Epidemiology*. Lippincott, Williams and Wilkins, Philadelphia, PA, 2008.

22. K. J. Rothman, S. Greenland, and A. M. Walker. Concepts of interaction. *American Journal of Epidemiology*, 112:467–470, 1980.
23. P. Royston and W. Sauerbrei. Interactions between treatment and continuous covariates: A step toward individualizing therapy. *Journal of Clinical Oncology*, 26:1397–1399, 2008.
24. L. B. Saltz, S. Clarke, E. Diaz-Rubio, et al. Bevacizumab in combination with oxaliplatin-based chemotherapy as first-line therapy in metastatic colorectal cancer: a randomized phase III study. *Journal of Clinical Oncology*, 26:2013–2019, 2008.
25. J. M. Satagopan and A. Iasonos. Measuring differential treatment benefit across marker specic subgroups: the choice of outcome scale. Technical report, Memorial Sloan Kettering Cancer Center, 2016. under review.
26. J. M. Satagopan, A. Iasonos, and Q. Zhou. Prognostic and predictive values and statistical interactions in the era of targeted treatment. *Genetic Epidemiology*, 39:509–517, 2015.
27. J. M. Satagopan, S. H. Olson, and R. C. Elston. Statistical interactions and Bayes estimation of log odds. *Statistical Methods in Medical Research*, 26:1021–1038, 2015. doi: 10.1177/0962280214567140.
28. J. M. Satagopan, A. Sen, Q. Zhou, et al. Bayes and empirical Bayes methods for reduced rank regression in matched case-control studies. *Biometrics*, 72:584–595, 2016.
29. J. M. Satagopan and R. C. Elston. Evaluation of removable statistical interaction for binary traits. *Statistics in Medicine*, 32:1164–1190, 2013.
30. C. L. Sawyers. The cancer biomarker problem. *Nature*, 452:548–552, 2008.
31. H. Scheffe. *The Analysis of Variance*. Wiley, New York, 1959.
32. S. E. Taube, G. M. Clark, J. E. Dancey, et al. A perspective on challenges and issues in biomarker development and drug and biomarker codevelopment. *Journal of the National Cancer Institute*, 101:1453–1463, 2009.
33. The Cancer Genome Atlas Research Network. Comprehensive genomic characterization defines human glioblastoma genes and core pathways. *Nature*, 455:1061–1068, 2008.
34. X. Wang, R. C. Elston, and X. Zhu. The meaning of interaction. *Human Heredity*, 70:269–277, 2010.
35. X. Wang, R. C. Elston, and X. Zhu. Statistical interaction in human genetics: how should we model it if we are looking for biological interaction? *Nature Reviews Genetics*, 12:74, 2011.
36. S. Zheng, A. D. Cherniack, N. Dewal, et al. Comprehensive pan-genomic characterization of adrenocortical carcinoma. *Cancer Cell*, 29:723–726, 2016. PMCID: PMC4864952.
37. G. Y. Zou. On the estimation of additive interaction by use of the four- by-two table and beyond. *American Journal of Epidemiology*, 168:212–224, 2008.

5

Design Considerations for Phase II Oncology Clinical Trials

Jared C. Foster
National Cancer Institute

Jennifer Le-Rademacher and Sumithra J. Mandrekar
Mayo Clinic

CONTENTS

5.1 Introduction

In phase II trials, the primary goal is to get a better understanding of the safety and efficacy of an intervention to make a go/no-go decision to "definitively" test that intervention in a subsequent phase III trial. Because such trials are generally designed to establish preliminary evidence (rather than "final" proof) of efficacy, a more liberal significance level (e.g., a two-sided type I error of 10%–20%) is often used for the primary hypothesis. Secondary goals of phase II trials include identification of subsets of the study population most likely to benefit from treatment, further evaluate toxicity profiles, quality of life (QOL) assessment, and other correlative endpoints.[1]

Given the somewhat exploratory nature of phase II trials, the endpoints used to evaluate a particular intervention in the phase II setting tend to differ from those that would be used to evaluate the same intervention in the phase III setting. In particular, phase II cancer trials tend to use shorter term endpoints, such as response rate, disease control rate, progression-free survival (PFS), and disease-free survival (DFS) rates at predetermined time points, whereas phase III trials tend to use time-to-event endpoints such as overall survival, PFS, and DFS.[1] As mentioned earlier, phase II trials are used to determine whether or not an intervention should be further evaluated in the phase III setting. Therefore, making the selection of an appropriate endpoint in the phase II setting is critical. In fact, results of a recent study suggest that the likelihood of a drug ultimately receiving FDA approval once it has reached the phase III setting is only approximately 50%, and that, among drug programs that are suspended in the phase III setting, approximately 54% are suspended for efficacy reasons.[2] Thus, it is important that the phase II endpoint will be a strong surrogate for the corresponding phase III endpoint in order to derive meaningful conclusions at the end of the trial with regard to the go/no-go decisions. Roughly speaking, this means that, ideally, the observed treatment effect on the phase II endpoint (or surrogate) will be strongly indicative of what the observed treatment effect would be on the corresponding phase III endpoint. However, the ideal phase II endpoint varies, depending on the type and severity of disease, and on the type of treatment being evaluated, making the validation of potential surrogate endpoints challenging.[1]

The goal of this chapter is to describe study designs that are commonly used in phase II trials in oncology and to discuss when each of these might be relevant. With increased interest in biomarker-based studies in recent years, much of the chapter focuses on design considerations for these studies. This chapter is organized as follows: design considerations for single-arm versus randomized trials (Section 5.2); various biomarker-based designs (Section 5.3); and design considerations for immunotherapy trials (Section 5.4). The chapter ends with a brief summary and some general guidelines in Section 5.5.

5.2 Single-Arm Versus Randomized Trials

A single-arm trial is designed using a historical control for comparison—all patients receive the same intervention and results are generally compared to a historical control. Because all patients receive the same intervention and the historical control provides a "fixed" target, single-arm trials can often be adequately powered with a relatively small number of patients; however, because the control group does not actually take part in the study, the conclusions made based on the findings of single-arm trials are generally not as strong as those made based on randomized trials. More specifically, the major drawback of a historical control is that the outcome of interest will not usually be observed under the same or similar trial conditions or sometimes even within the same population or similar time period. Thus, it is generally very difficult to know with certainty if any differences in outcomes between those receiving the intervention on study and the historical control are due to the intervention, due to differences in the population and/or trial settings, due to improvement in standard of care over time, or simply a result of expecting to get better or worse due to the fact that patients receiving the intervention know they are participating in a clinical trial. Because of this, a randomized trial design should be considered whenever possible. These advantages and challenges also apply to parallel multi-arm studies, where the outcomes of patients in each arm are compared to the historical control.

A simple two-arm study includes one arm that receives the intervention of interest and a separate "control" arm that receives the control intervention (instead of a historical control). Because the control group is now experiencing the same trial conditions, the potential for misleading results due to differences in patient characteristics and/or trial settings between the intervention and control arms is reduced. Moreover, because both arms are participating in the same trial, this often helps to reduce the potential for observed differences between groups resulting from patients knowing they are participating in a trial; however, the extent to which all of this is possible depends heavily on the manner in which patients are assigned to the arms (specifically, randomized vs. non-randomized), as well as the patients' awareness of which intervention they are receiving. While including a control arm helps to ensure that the intervention and control groups experience similar trial settings, this alone does not guarantee that the two groups will be directly comparable. To help better ensure comparability, patients should be assigned to one of the study arms randomly. Though not guaranteed, particularly when the study only contains a very small number of patients, this ensures that the study arms have a similar mixture of patients (in terms of their characteristics), thereby reducing the potential for observed differences in outcomes across the arms due to the fact that patient characteristics differ across arms. Furthermore, when possible, the randomization is either single- or double- blind—patients or both patients and treating physicians are blinded to which arm they have been assigned to. This helps ensure that patients in each study arm have similar expectations, thus reducing the potential for observed differences in outcome between study arms due to differences in expectations, which could be present if patients and/or treating physicians are aware of the intervention being received.

Mandrekar and Sargent[3] provide a detailed description of randomized phase II designs, which is briefly summarized here. Randomized phase II designs can be broken down into three categories: (1) randomization to parallel non-comparative single-arm experimental regimens, each of which contains an independent decision rule, that is, the outcome of each arm is compared to a historical control; (2) randomized selection designs, which select the most promising experimental regimen among several similar experimental regimens without a strict control on the type I error rates;

and (3) randomized screening designs, which compare an experimental regimen to standard of care. Example schemas for these designs are shown in Figures 5.1–5.3. In studies with randomly assigned, parallel, noncomparative interventions, each individual treatment arm is structured as an independent phase II study with determination of "promising activity" based on a comparison against a historical control, and the arms have independent decision rules for determining whether or not the treatments are worthy of further consideration in a phase III trial (and also for early termination for futility). Though uncommon, such designs may be attractive in situations where there is a reliable early endpoint to demonstrate success (for example, tumor response) that is directly attributable to the experimental regimen in question (such as a single-agent trial). However, success in such a trial generally continues to dictate the need for a more thorough evaluation of those regimens that show promise in a phase IIb setting, with a direct comparison of safety and efficacy outcomes between the randomized arms.

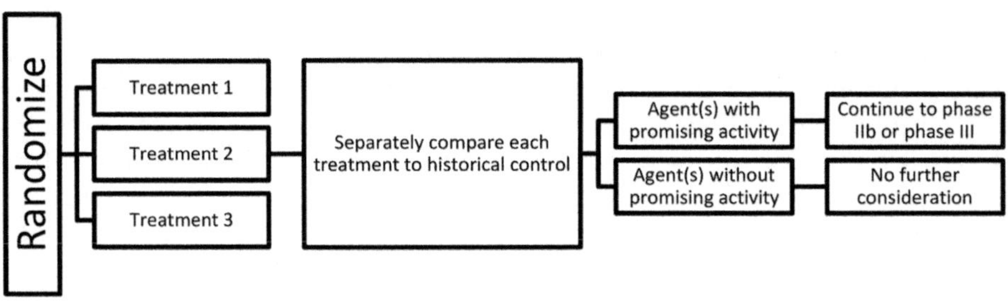

FIGURE 5.1
Three-arm, randomized, parallel non-comparative trial schema.

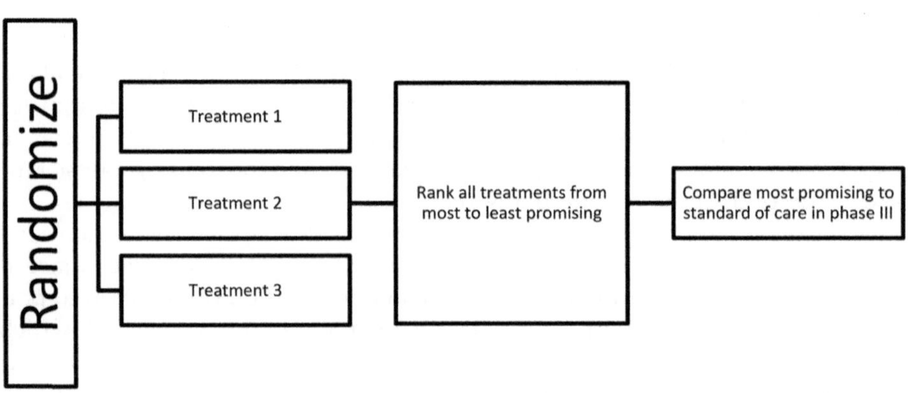

FIGURE 5.2
Three-arm, randomized selection design schema.

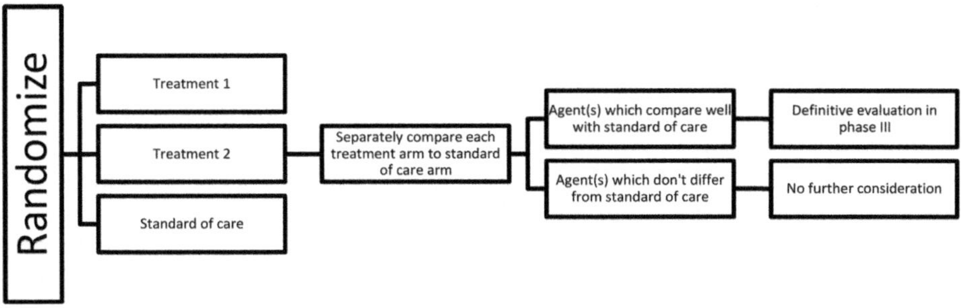

FIGURE 5.3
Three arm, randomized screening design schema.

The randomized selection design was first introduced by Simon et al.[4] With this type of design, the aim is to choose the most promising one among a number of experimental regimens (with no *a priori* data to suggest that one is superior to the others) using a ranking and selection approach, and the regimen(s) selected as the most promising is subsequently compared to the standard of care in a larger phase III trial. Such designs may be useful if, for example, one wishes to compare different modes of drug administration, different dosing schedules, or multiple combination regimens that have a new experimental agent added to a common core regimen. With selection designs, the sample size is determined by maximizing (as a function of study power, type-I error, and meaningful effect size) the probability of choosing the best arm (assuming one exists), assuming the expected outcome in that arm exceeds that of any other arm by a clinically meaningful margin (e.g., at least 15%). It is worth emphasizing that this design does not assess the relative merits of regimens, as it does not test the null hypothesis of equality of regimens.

In the randomized phase II setting, one may also wish to consider randomized screening designs, which involve the non-definitive comparison of one or more experimental regimes against the standard of care. This paradigm was formally introduced by Rubinstein et al.[5] to ensure both a high probability of identifying (and eliminating) non-promising and promising regimens for additional testing. It should be noted that these designs are not a replacement for a definitive phase III trial, but rather a tool, which may help to prioritize experimental regimens (using an intermediate endpoint) for a subsequent more definitive evaluation. With randomized screening designs, the power, type-I error, and target effect size must be selected carefully to ensure a reasonable sample size (and thus, meaningful results). If the type-I error (i.e., false-positive rate) is too large, one risks increasing the likelihood of the subsequent negative phase III trials. If the power is too low or the target effect size is too high, one risks terminating further testing of a potentially promising regimen. Rubinstein et al.[5] give a detailed discussion of potential choices for these parameters.

5.3 Biomarker-Based Phase II Designs

According to the Biomarkers Definitions Working Group, a biomarker is "a characteristic that is objectively measured and evaluated as an indicator of normal biological processes, pathogenic processes, or pharmacologic responses to a therapeutic intervention."[6] In oncology, the term biomarker refers to a broad range of measures, including those derived from tumor tissues, whole blood, plasma, serum, bone marrow, or urine.[7] Biomarkers are generally described as being either predictive or prognostic (or both), with the ultimate intended usage determining definition and the required validation methods.[7] Roughly speaking, a predictive marker is one that can be effectively used to guide treatment selection. More specifically, the predictive utility of a marker is determined by the extent to which the marker interacts with treatment, that is, the extent to which the expected response to a particular treatment varies across levels of the biomarker. In contrast, a prognostic marker is one that can be used to predict a patient's expected outcome, regardless of treatment (i.e., the "prognosis"). In this chapter, we focus primarily on predictive markers.

If there is strong evidence that a biomarker is predictive, and in particular, that the experimental treatment will only benefit certain marker-defined subpopulations, one may wish to consider an enrichment design in which patients are screened for one or more biomarkers, and only those in certain marker-defined subpopulations (specifically the subpopulations that are expected to respond well) are included in the trial.[8] The goal with a phase II enrichment design is to better understand the safety, tolerability, and clinical benefit of the experimental treatment in specific marker-defined subgroups.[9] A well-known example of this type of biomarker is the estrogen receptor (ER) status (predictive of response to endocrine therapy for breast cancer), as ER-positive tumors have been shown very likely to respond to endocrine therapy, whereas ER-negative tumors are unlikely to respond to such therapy.[10]

Sometimes, there may be preliminary evidence that a marker-defined subpopulation will respond well to an experimental treatment, but not enough evidence to rule out a positive response in patients outside this subpopulation. What this essentially means is that the predictive utility of the biomarker has not yet been confirmed. In such situations, one may wish to consider an all-comers design rather than an enrichment design. As the name suggests, an all-comers design allows for the enrolment of any eligible patient, regardless of biomarker status (though marker status is still measured). These designs generally involve an overall assessment of the treatment as well as prespecified subgroup analyses within marker-defined subpopulations, thus decreasing the risk of falsely concluding the experimental treatment to be ineffective in situations where it is only effective for a small, marker-defined subgroup of the population.[9]

One example of an all-comers design is that proposed by Friedlin et al.,[11] which could be considered for determining whether or not to assess experimental treatment in the phase III setting and whether or not the biomarker is truly predictive. Briefly speaking, in this design, patients are randomly assigned to either the experimental or control arms, and their marker status (either positive or negative) is recorded. Next, efficacy is assessed in the marker-positive patients and based on these results, additional analyses are performed using either the marker-negative patients or the entire study cohort. On the basis of the results of these analyses, one of the following decisions is made—to proceed to phase III using only marker-positive patients (i.e., phase III enrichment design), using a marker-stratified design, to proceed without the biomarker, or to not proceed to phase III at all. A schematic of this design is shown in Figure 5.4 to better illustrate the specific analyses and how each particular decision may be reached.

In our discussion of enrichment and all-comers designs, we have focused on the predictive nature of a biomarker and the degree to which its predictive utility has been established; however, these are only a few of the many factors to be considered when deciding between these two types of designs in the phase II setting. Other factors that may be of interest are the prevalence of the biomarker and the amount of time required to determine a patient's biomarker status.[9] Mandrekar and Sargent[9] provide a more in-depth discussion of this topic.

In our discussion of biomarker-based designs, we have thus far focused primarily on situations in which there are essentially two biomarker profiles of interest; however, there are many situations where more than two biomarker profiles are of interest. Furthermore, to this point, we have focused primarily on situations in which there is interest in evaluating the effect of an experimental regimen on a specific disease or histology, but in many situations, there may be evidence to suggest that an experimental treatment

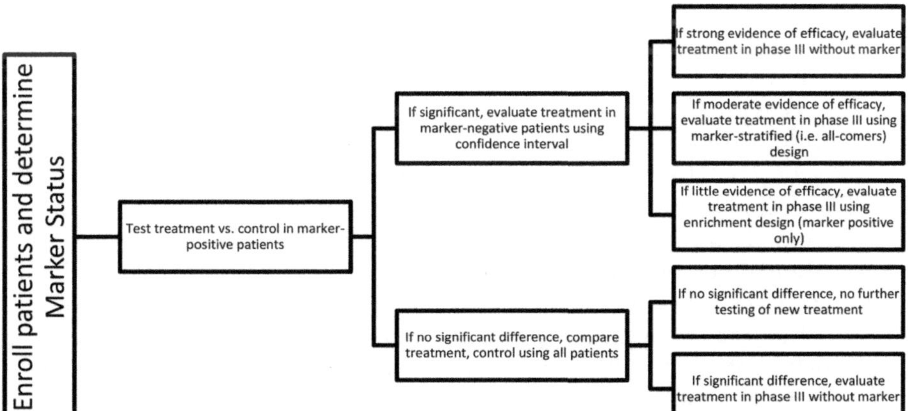

FIGURE 5.4
Friedlin et al. design schema.

may be effective across a variety of histologies, or even a variety of primary tumor sites. To this end, newer trial designs, namely, umbrella and basket designs, have been proposed in recent years to evaluate the effect of experimental regimens simultaneously on multiple biomarker-defined subpopulations for the same disease or histology (umbrella trial) or to evaluate the effect of a regimen on a biomarker-defined subpopulation simultaneously on multiple diseases/histology (basket trial). An umbrella trial or a basket trial consists of a master protocol with multiple sub-studies that can have the same design or different designs. Menis et al. provide a good review of these trial designs.[12] Description and examples of trials using these designs are given in the next sections.

5.3.1 Umbrella Trials

In umbrella trials, patients with a specific disease/histology are first screened for a set of targeted biomarkers and divided into biomarker-defined subpopulations (Figure 5.5a). Within each of these marker-defined subpopulations, a sub-study is then performed, with patients being assigned to a particular treatment as specified in the sub-study protocol. Patients who do not harbor any targeted biomarkers are either excluded from the trial or are enrolled in a no-abnormality subpopulation, and assigned to treatment as specified in the study. In the context of Phase II trials, the sub-studies within each master protocol can be of the designs described in Section 5.2 (single-arm, multiple-arm parallel, or multi-arm randomized trial). Examples of phase II umbrella trials include:

- BATTLE (Biomarker-integrated approaches of targeted therapy for lung cancer elimination) was a randomized, biomarker-based, phase II trial for patients with chemorefractory non–small cell lung cancer (NSCLC).[13] The design of this study was based on the evaluation of four different treatments for NSCLC (erlotinib, vandetanib, erlotinib+bexarotene, and sorafenib) with respect to the patient's response to one or more of these agents depending on his or her biomarker profile. In particular, the biomarker profiles of interest in this study were *EGFR, KRAS* or *BRAF, VEGF* or *VEGFR-2, RXR,* and/or *Cyclin D1.* This study utilized an adaptive randomization scheme, meaning the probability of a new patient being randomized to a particular treatment varied over the course of the study. In particular, patients who enrolled early in the study were randomly assigned to one of the four treatments with equal probability. However, randomization was weighted for patients who enrolled later in the study, such that each new patient was most likely to be randomized to the treatment that was expected to benefit him the most, based on the cumulative response data of patients with whom he shared a biomarker profile.[14] This type of randomization is referred to as outcome-adaptive randomization, as the randomization probability

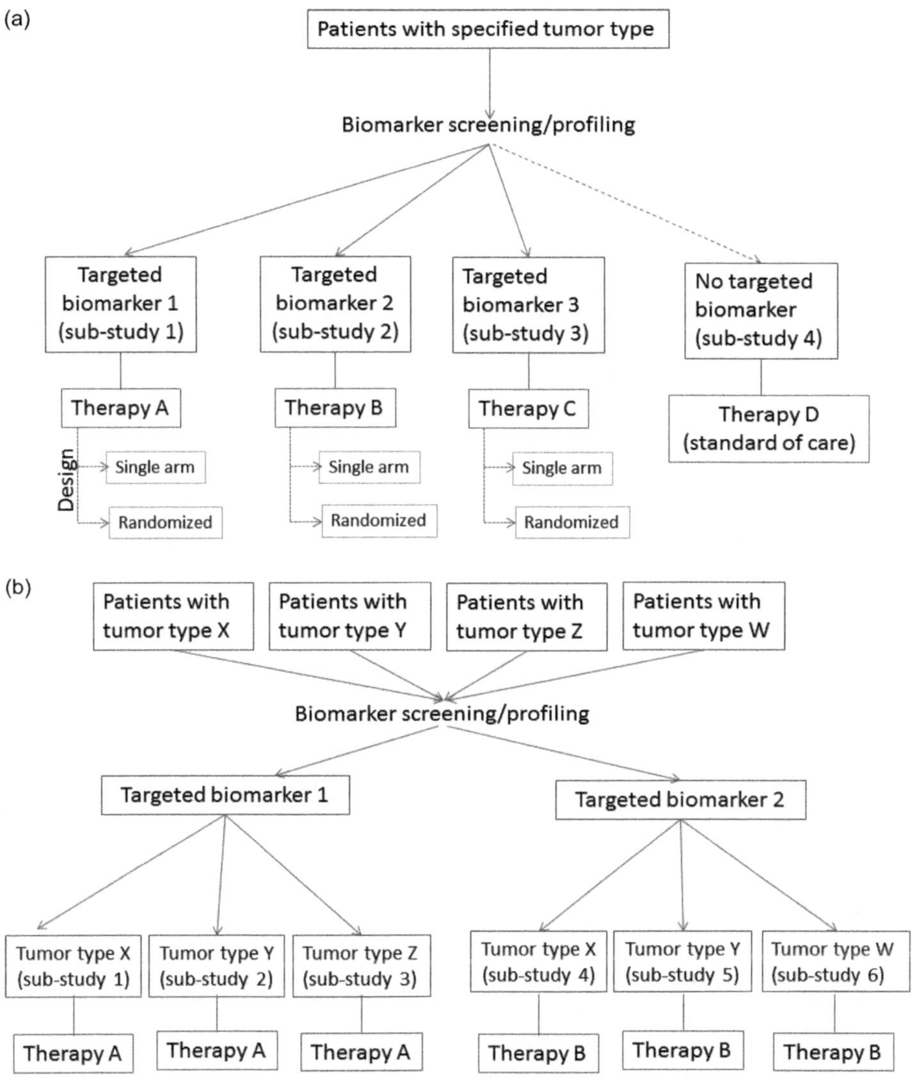

FIGURE 5.5
(a) Umbrella-trial schema (b) Basket-trial schema.

is based on the outcome by the biomarker subpopulation. This design allowed the study investigators to perform an overall evaluation of the four experimental regimens, as well as exploratory evaluation of the degree to which the response to a particular regimen varied across biomarker profiles.[13]

- BATTLE 2 (Biomarker-integrated targeted therapy study in previously treated patients with advanced NSCLC) was a randomized, biomarker-based, phase II trial for patients with advanced NSCLC (excluding sensitizing *EGFR* mutations and *ALK* gene fusions) refractory to more than one prior therapy, which employed a similar design to the BATTLE trial.[15] In this study, the targeted biomarker was *KRAS* mutation, and the four regimens tested were erlotinib, erlotinib+MK-2206, MK-2206+AZD6244, and sorafenib. This trial utilized an outcome-adaptive randomization scheme similar to that described for the BATTLE trial.

- SAFIR02-Lung (Evaluation of the efficacy of high throughput genome analysis as a therapeutic decision tool for patients with metastatic NSCLC) is an ongoing trial in which patients are screened for six target biomarkers and subsequently classified into biomarker subgroups.[16] The (prespecified) targeted therapies in this trial include AD2014 for *m-TOR*, AZD4547 for *FGFR*, AZD5363 for *AKT*, AZD8931 for *HER2/EGFR*, selumetinib for *MEK*, and Vandetanib for *VEGF/EGFR*. Patients in each biomarker group are randomized at a 2:1 ratio to the corresponding targeted therapy or standard maintenance therapy (erlotinib for squamous NSCLC or pemetrexed for non-squamous NSCLC). Those without targeted biomarkers are grouped into a separate subpopulation and randomized at a 2:1 ratio to either immunotherapy maintenance with MEDI4736 or standard maintenance therapy (same as the other sub-studies).

5.3.2 Basket Trials

Like umbrella designs, basket trials generally involve several biomarker profiles, across which the average response to one or more experimental treatments is expected to vary. However, while umbrella trials focus on a specific disease or histology, patients with a variety of tumor types and/or histologies are considered in basket trials. These designs may be appropriate when there is a reason to believe that one or more experimental treatments may be effective across a range of primary tumor sites or histologies, and in particular, when patients with specific biomarker profiles are expected to respond well to a particular treatment, regardless of their specific disease or histology. Thus, in basket trials, patients of several tumor types and/or histologies are screened for one or more biomarkers, and patients with the desired biomarker profiles are enrolled in the trial and divided by disease cohort (Figure 5.5b). Because of this, basket trials often consist of a collection of parallel phase II trials. Examples of Phase II basket trials include:

- CUSTOM (Molecular profiling and targeted therapies in advanced thoracic malignancies) enrolled patients with advanced NSCLC, small cell lung cancer, and thymic malignancies.[17] This study included five targeted therapies and several biomarker profiles. Specifically, the targeted therapies were erlotinib for *EGFR* mutations, selumetinib for *KRAS, HRAS, NRAS,* or *BRAF* mutations,

MK2206 for *PIK3CA, AKT*1, or *PTEN* mutations, lapatinib for *HER*2 mutations, and sunitinib for *KIT* or *PDGFRA* mutations. The study was designed to evaluate each treatment in all three histologic subtypes, for a total of 15 sub-studies, and each sub-study followed an optimal two-stage design. As noted by the study investigator, the goal of this study was "to identify molecular biomarkers and determine their frequency and clinical relevance in patients with advanced NSCLC, small cell lung cancer, and thymic malignancies, and to evaluate the efficacy of multiple targeted therapies in specific molecular subsets of patients."[17]

- CREATE (Cross-tumoral Phase II with crizotinib) is an ongoing trial for patients with locally advanced and/or metastatic anaplastic large cell lymphoma, inflammatory myofibroblastic tumor, papillary renal cell carcinoma type 1, clear cell sarcoma, alveolar soft part sarcoma, and alveolar rhabdomyosarcoma.[18] The targeted therapy of interest in this trial is crizotinib for *ALK* and/or *MET* alterations. In this case, the primary aim is "to study the antitumor activity of crizotinib across predefined tumor types in patients whose tumors are harboring specific alterations in ALK and/or MET."[18] The trial was designed as a parallel phase II trial with a separate arm for each of the six disease groups mentioned.
- NCI-MATCH (National Cancer InstituteMolecular analysis for therapy choice) is a large ongoing phase II trial enrolling patients with advanced solid tumors, lymphoma, and myeloma, with the goal of screening 5,000 patients.[19] The study currently targets 24 biomarkers with 16 different therapies. Briefly speaking, this trial "studies how well treatment that is directed by genetic testing works in patients with solid tumors or lymphomas that have progressed following at least one line of standard treatment or for which no agreed-upon treatment approach exists."[19] In this case, the investigators believe that patients with one of a number of genetic abnormalities may benefit more from the treatment that targets that abnormality.[19]

The basket-type trial design has also been used outside of the typical drug discovery setting. The French National Cancer Institute's AcSé (Secured Access to Innovative Therapies) initiative[20] and the American Society of Clinical Oncology (ASCO)'s Targeted agent and profiling utilization registry (TAPUR)[21] are examples of large-scale trials with basket-type design that evaluate the safety and efficacy profile of *approved* agents in other indications, that is, tumor types. The goals of these trials are to provide patients with advanced diseases (without promising treatment options) off-label access to approved agents and to evaluate the safety and efficacy of these agents outside of their approved indications. Similar to other basket trials, patients with various tumor types and/or histologies are first screened for one or more biomarkers. They are then given the agent that has been approved for other indications targeting the same biomarker they harbor. More information about these studies is as follows.

- AcSé—Crizotinib (Phase 2 study assessing efficacy and safety of crizotinib in patients harboring an alteration on *ALK, MET,* or *ROS*1). This is the first trial coordinated by the AcSé Program.[20] It includes patients with various solid and hematologic malignancies.[22] The study includes a total of 23 cohorts of disease and biomarker combinations and the targeted therapy is crizotinib for *ALK, MET,* or *ROS*1 alterations. In each of the 23 disease types, each sub-study is designed as a single-arm two-stage phase II trial, with a maximum cohort size varying from 20 to 37 evaluable patients.[20]
- TAPUR is the first clinical trial coordinated by ASCO. This study includes patients with non-Hodgkin lymphoma, multiple myeloma, advanced solid tumors, and various biomarker profiles. The study currently includes 15 targeted therapies.[23] Each sub-study is designed as a single-arm two-stage trial with a maximum cohort size of 28 evaluable patients.[24]

Recall that in basket trials, the targeted experimental treatment is determined based on the biomarker profile, rather than the specific disease or histology, and thus the same targeted therapy may be evaluated (in parallel sub-trials) in patients with a variety of histologies. Thus, though the targeted experimental agent may be the same across several sub-studies, the best design for each sub-study will depend on the specific disease or histology being considered. Note that each of these are now small phase II studies and thus the design considerations discussed earlier in this chapter may be useful in making these decisions. If only modest accrual is expected for one or more of the histologies considered within the trial, one may wish to evaluate (relative to some historical control) the biomarker-targeted experimental agents using single-arm sub-studies for these histologic groups. For histologies with higher anticipated accrual, it may be better to consider randomizing patients in these sub-studies to either the biomarker-targeted experimental therapy or some standard of care. Recently, some authors have also developed designs specifically for basket-type trials. One such design is the Bayesian basket design.[25] In this design, a Bayesian approach is used to model the response probabilities for the various histologic strata and two hypotheses are considered: (1) the response probabilities for a particular targeted agent are equal across the corresponding histologic strata, and (2) the activity of the drug is independent across these strata.[25] Every time a new patient's response is evaluated, the estimated posterior response probabilities from the Bayesian model are updated based on this observed response. With this design, one may wish to consider including one or more interim analyses at prespecified time points. In each of these interim analyses, the posterior response probabilities are estimated for each histologic stratum, and those for which the response probabilities are very small (or large) may be closed due to futility (or strong evidence of efficacy).[25] Once the trial is complete, final estimates of the posterior response probabilities in each histologic cohort can be obtained, and one can determine whether or not to further evaluate the targeted agent(s) of interest in one or more histologic strata in a subsequent, larger trial.

The trials used as examples above illustrate the many design variations of umbrella and basket trials. Of the umbrella trials, BATTLE and BATTLE2 are biomarker-based response-adaptive randomized trials, whereas the design of SAFIRE02-Lung resembles a typical umbrella trial (as illustrated in Figure 5.5a) with randomized sub-studies. Of the basket-type trials, CUSTOM and AcSé consist of one-stage sub-studies, whereas CREATE and NCI-MATCH consist of two-stage sub-studies.

With the ability to evaluate the effect of therapies simultaneously on multiple biomarkers and diseases, umbrella and basket trial designs help accelerate the discovery process of targeted therapy. By following one master protocol with multiple sub-studies, these trial designs help increase the efficiency of the trial development process. For example, in the more traditional setting, where separate protocols are specified for each sub-study, the SAFIRE_02, CUSTOM, AcSé, and NCI-MATCH trials would have to go through the review/approval process 7 (for 7 subpopulations), 15, 23, and 24 times, respectively. This structure also allows investigators the flexibility to close or add a sub-study, as the study progresses without affecting other sub-studies within the same trial. For example, only 2 (NSCLC with *EGFR* mutations and NSCLC with *KRAS* or *BRAF* mutations) of the 15 sub-studies in the CUSTOM trial completed accruing, as the accrual was unsuccessful for the other 13 rare histologic subtypes. However, because the sub-studies were designed as independent trials, the investigators were able to analyze and publish the two sub-studies that successfully accrued patients.[17] Another example is the NCI-MATCH trial, which started with 10 sub-studies, and has been expanded to 24.[26] In addition to the advantages discussed here, one advantage specific to the basket trial design is that the effect of treatment can be evaluated across all disease/histology groups and also separately by disease/histology. This allows rare diseases to be included along with more common diseases that would otherwise not be studied in a more traditional trial setting due to slow accrual or lack of statistical power.

5.4 Immunotherapy

Immunotherapy is a treatment strategy that uses the patient's own immune system to fight cancer cells.[27,28,29] Two types of immunotherapeutics that have gained traction in recent years are cancer vaccines and immune checkpoint blockades. Unlike chemotherapy, which directly attacks cancer cells, thus allowing its effect on the tumor (tumor shrinkage) to be observed shortly after treatment, immunotherapy must first induce a response from the host's immune system, which then launches an attack on the cancer cells, thereby potentially resulting in a potential delayed response. Response to immunotherapy can be observed after a period of stable disease, or even after an initial period of tumor growth, or appearance of new lesions.[30] Due to these differences in immunotherapy response patterns, conventional response criteria, such as the response evaluation criteria in solid tumors and the World Health Organization criteria do not effectively capture objective tumor response to immunotherapy. Furthermore, due to the delayed response, a delayed separation of survival curves has been observed when comparing immunotherapy versus placebo. To better evaluate tumor response in this setting, Hoos et al.[30] suggested three novel endpoint considerations for immunotherapy trials. First, they recommended the use of assay harmonization to minimize biomarker variability among patients in multicenter trials. Second, they recommended a set of immune-related response criteria, using the percentage of change in tumor burden between assessment time points to define objective response to immune therapy. To address the issue of delayed separation in survival curves, their third recommendation is to use alternative methods, such as simulation or numerical integration, to estimate the number of events needed when designing an immunotherapy trial. Although existing infrastructure can support immunotherapy trials and the trial designs described in this chapter are appropriate in the phase II immunotherapy setting, appropriate endpoints must be considered when designing this type of trials in order to effectively assess response to treatment. Another challenge with immunotherapy is that it has shown great effectiveness in certain subsets of patients and little or no benefit in other subsets. This is an opportunity to conduct biomarker-based studies using the designs described in Section 5.3 to help identify subsets (i.e., evaluate potential predictive markers) of patients that would benefit from these treatments. Should they exist, such biomarkers could subsequently be used to better evaluate candidate immunotherapies in Phase II and III settings.

5.5 Discussion

In the phase II setting, the primary goal is to better understand the safety and efficacy of an intervention to determine whether or not the intervention should be further evaluated in a subsequent phase III trial. When attempting to make this determination, there are a wide range of potential designs, and the best design(s) for a particular situation will depend on a large number of factors, including anticipated accrual, the number of experimental agents, and the existence of one or more predictive biomarkers. If only modest accrual is expected, a single-arm trial could be considered, in which the experimental treatment is given to all patients, and the response is evaluated relative to some historical control. If accrual is not a concern, it may be better to consider a larger, randomized design. If one wishes to simultaneously evaluate multiple experimental agents to determine which, if any, should be further evaluated, randomized phase II selection or screening designs may be of interest. In the presence of one or more predictive biomarkers, one may wish to consider a biomarker-based design. In the setting of a particular disease or histology with a number of treatment options available with a specific biomarker profile, an umbrella design may be of interest. Similarly, if one believes that patients with a certain biomarker profile may respond well to a particular biomarker-targeted agent, regardless of their specific disease or histology, a basket-type design may be ideal.

When considering biomarker-based designs in the phase II setting, one should also consider the specific predictive nature of the biomarker(s) of interest. It is worth emphasizing that "predictive" only means that the expected response to treatment *differs* across one or more marker-defined subpopulations. The specific way in which the expected response differs may vary considerably. For instance, suppose we have three biomarkers (and that a patient can either be positive or negative), which we denote "X", "Y", and "Z," and an experimental treatment, which we refer to as treatment "A." Furthermore, suppose that for all three markers, marker-positive patients respond extremely well to treatment A, whereas marker-negative patients show a mild positive response, no response, and a strong negative response for markers X, Y, and Z, respectively. All three of these markers could be considered predictive, but the specific designs considered for each would likely vary in the phase II setting. In particular, some type of all-comers design would almost certainly be used for marker X, as all patients are expected to show some benefit from receiving treatment A. For marker Y, the design would likely depend on the degree to which Y is known to be predictive, with an all-comers design likely being selected if marker Y were "suspected" of being predictive and an enrichment design being selected if it were "known" to be predictive. For marker Z, the design likely wouldn't depend on the predictive utility being "known" vs. "suspected", since even preliminary evidence that treatment A *might* harm Z negative patients would likely lead investigators to select an enrichment design including only Z positive patients. When considering umbrella or basket designs, there are a number of practical issues that should be addressed. First, it should be noted that a strong collaboration among all parties involved is required to successfully conduct an umbrella or a basket trial. Additional challenges facing umbrella and basket trials are the heterogeneity of quality of the samples and the lack of consistency across local laboratories.[12,17] These problems could be minimized by using a central lab for all samples; however, using a central lab requires close coordination between clinical sites and the lab, which further complicates the collaborative efforts required to successfully implement these types of trials.

References

1. Mandrekar SJ, Redman MW, and Billingham LJ. Clinical Trial Methodology in Lung Cancer: Study Design and End-Point Considerations. *IASLC Thoracic Oncology* (2nd edition). Eds. Ball DL, Scagliotti GV, and Pass HI, Elsevier, 2018, 620–627.
2. Hay M, Thomas DW, Craighead JL, Economides C, and Rosethal J. Clinical development success rates for investigational drugs. *Nature Biotechnology* 2014, 32: 40–51. doi:10.1038/nbt.2786.
3. Mandrekar SJ and Sargent DJ. Randomized phase II trials: Time for a new era in clinical trial design. *Journal of Thoracic Oncology : Official Publication of the International Association for the Study of Lung Cancer* 2010, 5(7): 932–934. doi:10.1097/JTO.0b013e3181e2eadf.
4. Simon R, Wittes RE, and Ellenberg SE. Randomized phase II clinical trials. *Cancer Treatment Reports* 1985, 69: 1375–1381.
5. Rubinstein LV, Korn EL, Freidlin B, Hunsberger S, Ivy SP, and Smith MA. Design issues of randomized phase II trials and a proposal for phase II screening trials. *Journal of Clinical Oncology* 2005, 23: 7199–7206.
6. Biomarkers Definitions Working Group. Biomarkers and surrogate endpoints: Preferred definitions and conceptual framework. *Clinical Pharmacology and Therapeutics* 2001, 69, 89–95.
7. Mandrekar S and Sargent D. Challenges of Using Predictive Biomarkers in Clinical Trials. In: *Design and Analysis of Clinical Trials for Predictive Medicine.* Eds. Matsui S, Buyse M, and Simon R, CRC Press, Mar 2015, 129–143.
8. Simon R and Maitournam A. Evaluating the efficiency of targeted designs for randomized clinical trials. *Clinical Cancer Research* October 15 2004, 10(20): 6759–6763. doi: 10.1158/1078–0432.CCR-04–0496.
9. Mandrekar SJ and Sargent DJ. All-comers versus enrichment design strategy in phase II trials. *Journal of Thoracic Oncology : Official Publication of the International Association for the Study of Lung Cancer* 2011, 6(4): 658–660. doi:10.1097/JTO.0b013e31820e17cb.
10. McShane LM, Hunsberger S, and Adjei AA. Effective incorporation of biomarkers into phase II trials. *Clinical Cancer Research : An Official Journal of the American Association for Cancer Research* 2009, 15(6): 1898–1905. doi:10.1158/1078–0432.CCR-08–2033.
11. Freidlin B, McShane LM, Polley MYC, and Korn EL. Randomized phase II trial designs with biomarkers. *Journal of Clinical Oncology* 2012, 30(26): 3304–3309. doi:10.1200/JCO.2012.43.3946.
12. Menis J, Hasan B, and Besse B. New clinical research strategies in thoracic oncology: clinical trial design, adaptive, basket and umbrella trials, new end-points

and new evaluations of response. *European Respiratory Review* 2014, 23(133): 367–378.
13. Kim ES, Herbst RS, Wistuba II, Lee, JJ, Blumenschein GR, Tsao A, Stewart DJ, Hicks ME, Erasmus J, Gupta S, and Alden, CM. The BATTLE trial: Personalizing therapy for lung cancer. *Cancer Discovery* 2011, 1(1): 44–53.
14. Zhou X, Liu S, Kim ES, Herbst RS, and Lee JJ. Bayesian adaptive design for targeted therapy development in lung cancer—a step toward personalized medicine. *Clinical Trials* 2008, 5(3): 181–193.
15. Papadimitrakopoulou V, Lee JJ, Wistuba II, Tsao AS, Fossella FV, Kalhor N, Gupta S, Byers LA, Izzo JG, Gettinger SN, Goldberg SB, Tang X, Miller VA, Skoulidis F, Gibbons DL, Shen L, Wei C, Diao L, Peng SA, Wang J, Tam AL, Coombes KR, Koo JS, Mauro DJ, Rubin EH, Heymach JV, Hong WK, and Herbst RS. The BATTLE-2 study: A biomarker-integrated targeted therapy study in previously treated patients with advanced non–small-cell lung cancer. *Journal of Clinical Oncology* 2016, 34(30): 3638–3647.
16. Clinicaltrials.gov. Evaluation of the Efficacy of High Throughput Genome Analysis as a Therapeutic Decision Tool for Patients with Metastatic Non-small Cell Lung Cancer. NCT02117167. https://clinicaltrials.gov/ct2/show/NCT02117167?term=safir02&rank=1. Date of last update: February 19, 2016.
17. Lopez-Chavez A, Thomas A, Rajan A, Raffeld M, Morrow B, Kelly R, Carter CA, Guha U, Killian K, Lau CC, Abdullaev Z, Xi L, Pack S, Meltzer PS, Corless CL, Sandler A, Beadling C, Warrick A, Liewehr DJ, Steinberg SM, Berman A, Doyle A, Szabo E, Wang Y, and Giaccone G. Molecular profiling and targeted therapy for advanced thoracic malignancies: A biomarker-derived, multiarm, multihistology phase II basket trial. *Journal of Clinical Oncology* 2015, 33(9): 1000–1007.
18. Cross-tumoral Phase 2 with Crizotinib. NCT 01524926. https://clinicaltrials.gov/ct2/show/study/NCT01524926?term=NCT01524926&rank=1. Date of last update: July 6, 2016.
19. NCI-MATCH: Targeted Therapy Directed by Genetic Testing in Treating Patients With Advanced Refractory Solid Tumors or Lymphomas. NCT 02465060. https://clinicaltrials.gov/ct2/show/record/NCT02465060. Date of last update: November 28, 2016.
20. Buzyn A, Blay J, Hoog-Labouret N, Jimenez M, Nowak F, Deley MC, Pérol D, Cailliot C, Raynaud J, and Vassal G. Equal access to innovative therapies and precision cancer care. *Nature Reviews – Clinical Oncology* 2016, 13: 385–393.
21. Brower V. American society of clinical oncology developing first clinical trial. *Journal of National Cancer Institute* 2015, 107: 3–4.
22. Phase 2 Study Assessing Efficacy and Safety of Crizotinib in Patients Harboring an Alteration on ALK, MET or ROS1 (AcSé). NCT 02034981. https://clinicaltrials.gov/ct2/show/record/NCT02034981?term=02034981&rank=1. Date of last update: February 16, 2016.
23. Clinicaltrials.gov. TAPUR: Testing the Use of Food and Drug Administration (FDA) Approved Drugs That Target a Specific Abnormality in a Tumor Gene in People With Advanced Stage Cancer (TAPUR). NCT02693535. https://clinicaltrials.gov/ct2/show/record/NCT02693535. Date of late update December 16, 2016.
24. http://www.tapur.org/sites/tapur.org/files/11.23.16_General_TAPUR_Study_Overview.pdf

25. Simon R, Geyer S, Subramanian J, and Roychowdhury S. The bayesian basket design for genomic variant-driven phase II trials. *Seminars in Oncology* 2016, 43: 13–18.
26. http://ecog-acrin.org/wp-content/uploads/materials/EAY131/NCI-MATCH-EAY131-Interim-Analysis-Executive-Summary.pdf.
27. Drake CG, Lipson EJ, and Brahmer JR. Breathing new life into immunotherapy: Review of melanoma, lung and kidney cancer. *Nature Reviews Clinical Oncology* 2014, 11: 24–37.
28. Rosenberg SA, Yang JC, and Restifo NP. Cancer immunotherapy: Moving beyond current Vaccines. *Nature Medicine* 2004, 10: 909–915.
29. Mellman I, Coukos G, and Dranoff G. Cancer immunotherapy comes of age. *Nature Review* 2011, 480: 480–489.
30. Hoos A, Eggermont, AMM, Janetzki S, Hodi FS, Ibrahim R, Anderson A, Humphrey R, Blumenstein B, Old L, and Wolchok J. Improved endpoints for cancer immunotherapy trials. *JNCI* 2010, 102: 1388–1397.

6

Precision Medicine and Associated Challenges

Rajesh Talluri
The University of Mississippi Medical Center

Sanjay S. Shete
The University of Texas MD Anderson Cancer Center

CONTENTS

6.1 Introduction

Precision medicine refers to the use of genetic, environmental, and clinical information of a particular patient to tailor the treatment being administered to that patient [1]. Traditional clinical trials have been integral to the discovery of drugs to combat various diseases [2]; however, they often take a decade to complete and require thousands of participants, which are not desirable characteristics for clinical trials in precision medicine. As our understanding of human biology increases, we have enormous amounts of data of different types, such as DNA sequencing, methylation, protein expression, and imaging to help us better understand a disease. Collecting several different types of data in a clinical trial and borrowing strength from them would lead to the design of better clinical trials that take less time to complete and have higher success rates.

Precision medicine has already started impacting many areas of medical practice and disease prevention. Genetic testing for *BRCA1/BRCA2* mutations has been incorporated into routine cancer screening and plays an important role in breast cancer prevention [3,4]. Furthermore, a study analyzing clinical trials for drug development in breast cancer found that the success rate of trials increased when patients were selected for a trial based on the status of human epidermal growth factor receptor 2 (HER2) [5]. A similar study of clinical trials for non–small cell lung cancer (NSCLC) showed that biomarker-targeted therapies were six times more likely to succeed compared to traditional clinical trials [6].

Over the past few years, several methodologies have emerged to address the growing need for a new approach to clinical trials. In this chapter, we focus on examples of Bayesian adaptive trial designs. We discuss challenges associated with implementing these clinical trials, such as tumor heterogeneity and the use of different types of omic data.

6.2 Adaptive Bayesian Clinical Trials

In a clinical trial, there is generally some amount of prior information about the drug/treatment that is being tested in the trial. Applying traditional frequentist statistical methods, this information is used in the design of the trial but not in the analysis. Bayesian statistics provides a mathematical tool to calculate the likelihood of an event based on prior information. Suppose the parameter of interest in the trial is θ (e.g., the efficacy of a treatment). Then, the prior probability distribution, prior(θ), is the information about θ that was obtained from previous pilot studies or previous clinical trials. The likelihood function, lik(data$|\theta$), describes the likelihood of observing the current data observed in the current clinical trial given the parameter θ. Our main interest in this trial is to understand the distribution of θ. This can be accomplished using Bayes' theorem by combining the prior information and likelihood information to compute the posterior distribution of θ,

$$\text{posterior}(\theta|\text{data}) = \text{lik}(\text{data}|\theta) \times \text{prior}(\theta)\text{prob}(\text{data}).$$

This is a practical way of analyzing clinical trials, as typically participants are sequentially enrolled in the clinical trial in groups. Furthermore, if the clinical trial is performed in multiple stages, the information from previous stages can be used as prior information for the next stage, thereby possibly improving the assignment of the patients to the optimal treatment arm. Bayesian clinical trials are very flexible and naturally adaptive [7]. Adaptations such as dropping a treatment in the trial that has a low probability of success or adding a new treatment can be naturally incorporated in a Bayesian clinical trial design [8,9]. Also, a Bayesian clinical trial design allows for controlling for multiple responses in a clinical trial. One of the more practical and interesting aspects of Bayesian clinical trials is that patients can be assigned adaptively to treatments based on the success rate of the treatments in the trial, so that the patients participating in the trial are more likely to receive a superior treatment and are exposed to fewer risks [10,11]. These trials can be evaluated continuously and can output information to decide whether the trial is going to be successful or not at different stages of the trial.

There are many different types of Bayesian trial designs depending on the type of trial and the questions that need to be answered. There may also be trials for which adaptive randomization is not preferable [12]. Here, we perform case studies for two trials, the BATTLE and the I-SPY clinical trials.

6.3 Case Studies of Clinical trials

6.3.1 BATTLE Trial

The Biomarker-integrated approaches of targeted therapy for lung cancer elimination (BATTLE-1) program of personalized medicine (ClinicalTrials.gov numbers: NCT00409968, NCT00411671, NCT00411632, NCT00410059, and NCT00410189) is a novel phase II clinical trial that was designed based on adaptive randomization of patients using tumor markers. Tumor biomarkers play an important role in determining the treatment for patients with NSCLC because patients with mutations of the epidermal growth factor receptor (EGFR) experience improved outcomes with EGFR tyrosine kinase inhibitors.

The BATTLE-1 trial consisted of an umbrella protocol that included four parallel phase II trials for patients with advanced NSCLC who had been previously treated with chemotherapy and subsequently experienced disease relapse. The four treatment arms under the umbrella protocol used erlotinib (target: EGFR), sorafenib (target: KRAS/BRAF), bexarotene and erlotinib (target: retinoid-EGFR signaling), and vandetanib (target: vascular endothelial growth factor receptor [VEGFR]) to target the selected gene pathways. The motivation for the trial design was to assign patients with certain biomarker profiles to matching treatments with agents that target the pathways corresponding to those biomarkers and thereby providing personalized treatment for the patients enrolled in the study.

Initially, under the umbrella protocol, the patients enrolled in the study underwent tissue biopsy for biomarker analysis. The treatment to which a patient was assigned was then determined according to the patient's biomarker profile, which was based on 11 biomarkers: *EGFR* mutation, *EGFR* overexpression/amplification, *EGFR* increased copy number (in the *EGFR* pathway), *KRAS* mutation, *BRAF* mutation (in the *KRAS/BRAF* pathway), *VEGFR* expression, *VEGFR-2* expression (in the *VEGFR* pathway), *RXRα* expression, *RXRβ* expression, *RXRγ* expression, and cyclin D1 expression (in the *RXR*/cyclin D1 pathway). Classifying patients based on 11 biomarkers leads to 2,048 (2^{11}) possible groups. To reduce the complexity of the trial, the number of possible groups was reduced to 5 based on certain predefined biomarker profiles: 1) *EGFR* pathways are positive; 2) *KRAS* or *BRAF* mutations; 3) VEGF and/or VEGF-2 overexpression; 4) RXRs α, β, and γ, and/or cyclin D1 overexpression and/or *CCND1* amplification; or 5) missing or incomplete biomarker information. In comparison to a traditional single-arm clinical trial that encompasses one study, this clinical trial implemented 20 parallel studies to evaluate the primary endpoints for individuals with five biomarker profiles who were assigned to four treatment groups.

The primary endpoint used to evaluate the study was the 8-week disease control rate (DCR), which is defined as the percentage of patients that have achieved complete response, partial response, and stable disease status following the therapeutic interventions in the trial [13]. To evaluate the endpoints for each of the four treatment options and five patient groups, a Bayesian probit model [14] was used to identify the best treatment for each group of patients. Let DCR_{ijk} denote the DCR for patient *i* assigned to the treatment option *j* in the biomarker group *k*. The Bayesian probit model can be specified as shown below using a random variable Z_{ijk} that signifies disease progression and a latent variable γ_{ijk}:

$$\mathrm{DCR}_{ijk} = P\left(Z_{ijk} = 1\right)$$

$$Z_{ijk} = \begin{cases} 0 \text{ if } \gamma_{ijk} \le 0 \\ 1 \text{ if } \gamma_{ijk} > 0 \end{cases}$$

$$\gamma_{ijk} \sim N\left(\mu_{jk}, 1\right)$$

$$\mu_{jk} \sim N\left(\alpha_j, \sigma^2\right)$$

$$\alpha_j \sim N\left(0, \tau^2\right),$$

where γ_{ijk} has a normal prior with parameters that in turn have normal hyperpriors. This model allows for borrowing information across the different treatment and biomarker groups. For each patient, the probability of randomization to treatment group *j* can be computed from the posterior distribution of this model as $\frac{\widehat{\mathrm{DCR}}_{jk}}{\sum_{j \in J} \widehat{\mathrm{DCR}}_{jk}}$, where $\widehat{\mathrm{DCR}}_{jk}$ is the posterior mean.

At the start of the study, the randomization of patients was uniform for all the four treatment groups. The goal was to evaluate the study periodically as patients were enrolled in the study and use adaptive randomization to assign new patients to treatments based on the biomarker profiles that were associated with better primary endpoints for the treatment options. The BATTLE trial was continuously assessed and followed termination rules that would drop treatments early for findings of futility for each of the five biomarker profiles. The stopping rule was that if the likelihood of DCR > 50% was less than 10% for a treatment–biomarker profile combination, the corresponding treatment was suspended for that biomarker profile. The primary hypothesis for a treatment–biomarker profile combination to be promising was to have the likelihood of DCR > 30% to be at least 80%. To have higher power for detecting promising treatments and low probability of missing potentially promising treatments, a higher type 1 error rate was used in the study.

The study was conducted on 341 participants with NSCLC. Initially, 97 patients were randomly assigned to the treatments, and 158 patients were adaptively randomized based on the posterior probabilities. The remaining 86 patients had specific conditions that prevented them from being randomly assigned to a treatment. At the end of the study, data from 244 patients were used for the analysis. The 8-week DCR was 46% for the whole study, with the four treatments (erlotinib, sorafenib, bexarotene and erlotinib, and vandetanib) having respective DCRs of 34%, 58%, 50%, and 33%. Eight combinations of a treatment plus a biomarker profile were proven to be effective (likelihood of DCR > 30% is at least 80%) at the end of the study.—Those are

1. erlotinib in the group with VEGF and/or VEGF-2 overexpression;
2. vandetanib in the group with EGFR pathways positive;
3. erlotinib plus bexarotene in the group with EGFR pathways positive;
4. erlotinib plus bexarotene in the group with RXRs α, β, and γ, and/or cyclin D1 overexpression;
5. erlotinib plus bexarotene in the group with missing or incomplete biomarker information;
6. sorafenib in groups with *KRAS* or *BRAF* mutation;
7. sorafenib in groups with VEGF and/or VEGF-2 overexpression;
8. sorafenib in groups with missing or incomplete biomarker information.

This trial confirmed the feasibility of using biomarker-based trials to achieve better disease control and paved the way for clinical trials based on precision medicine [15]. One of the limitations of the BATTLE-1 trial was that the biomarker profiles were bundled into five predefined groups to reduce the complexity of the trial, which may not be the optimal way to group individuals with different biomarker profiles. At the end of the study, some of the selected biomarkers had no predictive or prognostic values, which resulted in groups that had no relationship with a treatment. This decreased the statistical power of the study. Extensions to the trial have been proposed for selecting predictive markers using a two-stage adaptive Bayesian lasso approach [16]. This has led to the design of the BATTLE-2 trial [17], which uses a Bayesian two-stage biomarker-based adaptive randomization strategy. Biomarkers are selected in the first stage and validated in the second stage using a two-step Bayesian lasso model, which initially uses a group lasso to select biomarkers and an adaptive lasso to refine the selected biomarkers by assessing the predictive effect of the biomarkers from the trial.

The BATTLE-2 trial was also a phase II study that evaluated treatments for patients with advanced NSCLC. However, patients with *EML4-ALK* fusion or *EGFR* mutation were excluded from the BATTLE-2 study. *KRAS* mutation status was used as the stratifying factor for the participants in the first stage as the main goal was to evaluate therapies that targeted cancers related to *KRAS* mutations. Next-generation sequencing and gene expression profiling were performed on tumor biopsies to evaluate predictive and prognostic biomarkers. The participants were then randomized into one of the four treatment arms: (1) erlotinib, (2) erlotinib plus MK-2206, (3) MK-2206 plus AZD6244, or (4) sorafenib.

A total of 334 patients were recruited for the study, of which data from 186 patients were available for analysis at the end of the study. The remaining 148 patients were not included in the analysis because they either did not meet the eligibility criteria, declined to give their consent, or were unable to be randomized to a treatment in the trial because of certain conditions. Similar to the BATTLE-1 trial, the 8-week DCR was used as the primary endpoint for the trial. One of the major pitfalls for this trial was that none of the biomarkers was predictive for any of the four treatment arms. The BATTLE-2 trial was based on grouping patients with predictive or prognostic markers for each treatment into the treatment arm that was expected to provide them with the most benefit. Having no predictive markers for the treatment arms lowered the power of the trial, which did not discover any findings that were clinically relevant. Nevertheless, the BATTLE-2 study showcased the trial design for the utility of biomarkers for better target selection and treatment response to improve clinical care for patients enrolled in clinical trials.

6.3.2 I-SPY Trials

The investigation of serial studies to predict your therapeutic response with imaging and molecular analysis 2 (I-SPY 2) (ClinicalTrials.gov numbers: NCT01042379) is a phase II adaptive Bayesian clinical trial in the neoadjuvant setting for women with locally advanced breast cancer. I-SPY2 was developed to efficiently and quickly test drug–biomarker combinations for treating breast cancer and enable the development of more informed phase III trials.

The I-SPY 2 trial [18] was designed as a flexible trial that incorporates multiple biomarkers and multiple treatments. It aims to match patients' biomarker profiles to particular treatments that target their biomarker profiles or to particular treatments that have been shown to be effective for patients with similar profiles. Biomarkers are classified into three groups: 1) standard biomarkers approved by the Food and Drug Administration (FDA); 2) qualifying biomarkers that have not yet been approved by the FDA but which are promising and have sufficient existing data to confirm their viability; and 3) exploratory biomarkers that were derived from promising pilot studies and will be evaluated during the trial.

Patients are stratified into different groups using these biomarkers. The qualifying and experimental biomarkers are evaluated using sensitivity and specificity metrics for the accuracy of stratification of patients and are included in the trial if they meet the criterion for accuracy. Standard biomarkers, such as the estrogen receptor (ER+/–), progesterone receptor (PR+/–), HER2+/–, and MammaPrint score, are measured. Patients with low MammaPrint, ER-positive, and HER2-negative status are excluded from the trial because it has been shown that chemotherapy is not an ideal treatment for these patients.

I-SPY 2 was designed to evaluate the effectiveness of novel drugs in combination with standard chemotherapy compared to standard chemotherapy alone. The treatments found to have higher efficacy than the standard treatment successfully progress to the next stage, phase III trials; whereas those with lower efficacy than the standard treatment are dropped from the study. Each drug is tested on a minimum of 20 patients and a maximum of 120 patients before a decision is made regarding its efficacy. As the tested drugs move from the study, new drugs are accepted as additions to the study based on certain criteria such as known efficacy in breast cancer, compatibility with standard taxane therapy, the effect on key targets in breast cancer, and sufficient availability of the drug.

The I-SPY 2 trial has two control arms for standard chemotherapy and other arms that are used to test the efficacy of new drugs simultaneously. After stratification based on biomarker groups, a Bayesian adaptive randomization scheme [8] for a particular new drug is used to assign patients to one of the arms based on their biomarker profile. Drugs that perform better for patients with a particular biomarker profile show efficacy more quickly and proceed to the next stage as more individuals with that particular profile are assigned to that treatment based on the posterior probabilities.

The I-SPY 2 trial provides a very sophisticated framework for the development of clinical trials for precision medicine. Many pharmaceutical and biotechnological companies are participating in this trial, which is disseminating an enormous amount of knowledge and advancing science at a faster rate to improve our understanding of the disease.

6.4 Challenges in the Implementation of Precision Medicine Trials

The first step in precision medicine trials is to perform some sort of biological sample analysis to evaluate the molecular or biomarker profile of the participants enrolling in the study. This provides a host of challenges to ensure that the profiling procedure is the same for all participants. Some of the challenges arise because of heterogeneity and lack of standardization among the various platforms for biological analysis (e.g., next-generation sequencing, methylation, protein expression).

6.4.1 Heterogeneity in Biological Specimens

Heterogeneity is a very important issue in precision medicine trials as it is based on the classification of individuals into groups according to their biological profile. A biological analysis is carried out to ensure that what is being measured is a reliable basis for grouping individuals together. This is where heterogeneity plays a major role, as there are different types of heterogeneity. The simplest form of heterogeneity is population heterogeneity, which may arise because of covariates for each individual in the study such as race, smoking status, and body mass index. The trial investigators can account for these variations among the participants by incorporating them as covariates in the analytic model that is used to analyze the data from the trial.

A more complicated form of heterogeneity comes from biological specimens. These include the location from which the specimen is taken and how well the specimen can represent the biological profile of the patient. In cancer clinical studies, drugs are developed to target particular genetic mutations in the tumor. However, cancer is an evolving disease; hence, tumors are constantly responding to their environment by taking on different molecular characteristics [19]. When a biological sample is excised from a tumor, its molecular profile may not reveal the whole biological profile of the disease; therefore, a treatment matched to that profile may not be effective in killing all the tumor cells. Spatial heterogeneity in tumors gives rise to this type of issue because the specific location from which the tumor sample was taken may affect the tumor's response to a given treatment. Dealing with spatial heterogeneity would require taking multiple samples of the tumor from different locations, which is generally not recommended by clinicians due to the risks associated with a more invasive procedure [20]. In some cases, the location of a tumor within the body may render some tumor sites completely inaccessible for a tissue biopsy.

Another type of heterogeneity is temporal heterogeneity. As cancer is an evolving disease, a tumor may evolve such that it attains a very different biological signature that may allow it to evade the targeted treatment assigned to that particular biological profile at the start of the study. Hence, the targeted treatment will fail to be effective in individuals with cancer characterized by such temporal heterogeneity [21]. Furthermore, drug-resistant tumors may evolve in response to the effects of treatment on the tumor cells, which may be hard to evaluate in a clinical trial.

Dealing with temporal heterogeneity would require individuals to have repeated biological profiling at specific intervals in the study. This may not be feasible due to the risks associated with taking multiple tumor samples or due to the associated cost. For cancer types with circulating tumor cells, an alternative way of assessing temporal heterogeneity would be to obtain the circulating tumor cells from the blood instead of sampling tissues from the tumor [22]; however, the effectiveness of such an approach relative to accurate profiling has yet to be determined. Novel methods to model tumor heterogeneity and changes in tumor heterogeneity in response to treatment should be developed to account for these effects while analyzing data from precision medicine clinical trials.

Acknowledgments

Supported by the National Cancer Institute [P30CA016672 to S. Shete]; the Barnhart Family Distinguished Professorship in Targeted Therapy [to S. Shete]; The Duncan Family Institute for Cancer Prevention and Risk Assessment [to S. Shete]; and the Cancer Prevention Research Institute of Texas [grant RP170259 to S. Shete].

References

1. Lu YF, Goldstein DB, Angrist M, Cavalleri G. Personalized medicine and human genetic diversity. *Cold Spring Harbor Perspect Med.* 2014; 4(9): a008581–a008581.
2. Cohen MH, Williams G, Johnson JR, Duan J, Gobburu J, Rahman A, Benson K, Leighton J, Kim SK, Wood R, Rothmann M. Approval summary for imatinib mesylate capsules in the treatment of chronic myelogenous leukemia. *Clin Cancer Res.* 2002; 8(5): 935–942.
3. Domchek SM, Friebel TM, Singer CF, Evans DG, Lynch HT, Isaacs C, Garber JE, Neuhausen SL, Matloff E, Eeles R, Pichert G, Van t'veer L, Tung N, Weitzel JN, Couch FJ, Rubinstein WS, Ganz PA, Daly MB, Olopade OI, Tomlinson G, Schildkraut J, Blum JL, Rebbeck TR. Association of risk-reducing surgery in BRCA1 or BRCA2 mutation carriers with cancer risk and mortality. *J Am Med Assoc.* 2010; 304(9): 967–975.
4. Høberg-Vetti H, Bjorvatn C, Fiane BE, Aas T, Woie K, Espelid H, Rusken T, Eikesdal HP, Listøl W, Haavind MT, Knappskog PM, Haukanes BI, Steen VM, Hoogerbrugge N. BRCA1/2 testing in newly diagnosed breast and ovarian cancer patients without prior genetic counselling: The DNA-BONus study. *Eur J Hum Genet.* 2015; 24(6): 881–888.
5. Parker J, Lushina N, Bal P, Petrella T, Dent R, Lopes G. Impact of biomarkers on clinical trial risk in breast cancer. *Breast Cancer Res Treat.* 2012; 136(1):179–185.
6. Falconi A, Lopes G, Parker J. Biomarkers and receptor targeted therapies reduce clinical trial risk in non-small-cell lung cancer. *J Thoracic Oncol.* 2014; 9(2): 163–169.

7. Berry SM, Carlin BP, Jack Lee J. *Bayesian adaptive methods for clinical trials.* CRC Press, 2010.
8. Berry DA. Bayesian clinical trials. *Nature Rev Drug Disc* 2006; 5: 27–36.
9. Berry DA, Muss HB, Cirrincione CT, Theodoulou M, Mauer AM, Kornblith AB, Partridge AH, Dressler LG, Cohen HJ, Becker HP, Kartcheske PA, Wheeler JD, Perez EA, Wolff AC, Gralow JR, Burstein HJ, Mahmood AA, Magrinat G, Parker BA, Hart RD, Grenier D, Norton L, Hudis CA, Winer EP. Adjuvant chemotherapy in older women with early-stage breast cancer. *N Engl J Med.* 2009; 360: 2055–2065.
10. Thompson W. On the likelihood that one unknown probability exceeds another in view of the evidence of two samples. *Biometrika* 1933; 25: 285–294.
11. Meuer WJ, Lewis RJ, Berry DA. Adaptive clinical trials: A partial remedy for the therapeutic misconception? *J Am Med Assoc.* 2012; 307: 2377–2378.
12. Lee JJ, Chen N, Yin G. Worth adapting? Revisiting the usefulness of outcome-adaptive randomization. *Clin Cancer Res.* 2012; 18: 4498–4507.
13. Lara PN Jr, Redman MW, Kelly K, Edelman MJ, Williamson SK, Crowley JJ, Gandara DR. Disease control rate at 8 weeks predicts clinical benefit in advanced non-small-cell lung cancer: Results from Southwest Oncology Group randomized trials. *J Clin Oncol.* 2008; 26: 463–467.
14. Zhou X, Liu S, Kim ES, Herbst RS, Lee JJ. Bayesian adaptive design for targeted therapy development in lung cancer–a step toward personalized medicine. *Clin Trials.* 2008; 5: 181–193.
15. Lee JJ, Gu X, Liu S. Bayesian adaptive randomization designs for targeted agent development. *Clin Trials.* 2010; 7: 584–596.
16. Gu X, Yin G, Lee JJ. Bayesian two-step Lasso strategy for biomarker selection in personalized medicine development for time-to-event endpoints. *Contemp Clin Trials.* 2013; 36: 642–650.
17. Papadimitrakopoulou V, Lee JJ, Wistuba II, Tsao AS, Fossella FV, Kalhor N, Gupta S, Byers LA, Izzo JG, Gettinger SN, Goldberg SB, Tang X, Miller VA, Skoulidis F, Gibbons DL, Shen L, Wei C, Diao L, Peng SA, Wang J, Tam AL, Coombes KR, Koo JS, Mauro DJ, Rubin EH, Heymach JV, Hong WK, Herbst RS. The BATTLE-2 study: a biomarker-integrated targeted therapy study in previously treated patients with advanced non–small-cell lung cancer. *J Clin Oncol.* 2016; 34: 3638–3647.
18. Barker AD, Sigman CC, Kelloff GJ, Hylton NM, Berry DA, Esserman LJ. I-SPY 2: An adaptive breast cancer trial design in the setting of neoadjuvant chemotherapy. *Clin Pharmacol Ther.* 2009; 86(1): 97–100.
19. Meacham CE, Morrison SJ. Tumour heterogeneity and cancer cell plasticity. *Nature* 2013; 501(7467): 328–337.
20. Le Tourneau C, Kamal M, Alt M, Verlingue L, Servois V, Sablin MP, Servant N, Paoletti X. The spectrum of clinical trials aiming at personalizing medicine. *Chin Clin Oncol.* 2014; 3(2): 13.
21. Turner NC, Reis-Filho JS. Genetic heterogeneity and cancer drug resistance. *Lancet Oncol.* 2012; 13(4): e178–e185.
22. Pestrin M, Salvianti F, Galardi F, De Luca F, Turner N, Malorni L, Pazzagli M, Di Leo A, Pinzani P. Heterogeneity of PIK3CA mutational status at the single cell level in circulating tumor cells from metastatic breast cancer patients. *Mol Oncol.* 2015; 9(4): 749–757.

7

Use of Adaptive Design in Late-Stage Oncology Trials

Satrajit Roychoudhury
Pfizer Inc.

Arunava Chakravartty and Pabak Mukhopadhyay
Novartis Pharmaceutical Company

CONTENTS

7.1 Introduction

Adaptive designs play an increasingly important role in modern drug development. Such designs use accumulating data to decide how to modify the design of an ongoing trial without undermining the validity and integrity of the trial. Adaptive designs thus allow for a number of possible changes at midterm including early stopping for futility or success, sample size reassessment, dose selection, change of population, and so on. However, they require careful statistical and operational considerations. Historically, adaptive trials are widely in exploratory phases of drug development. In recent years, they have also gained popularity in the confirmatory setting [26] as drug makers and regulators are exploring ways to make the drug development process more efficient.

In 2010, the U.S. Food and Drug Administration (FDA) released guidance on adaptive designs in clinical trials [36]. This guidance discusses a wide range of adaptive designs used in clinical studies, including both familiar and less familiar approaches. In this chapter, we have focused on two specific types of adaptive designs mentioned in the FDA guidance. They are known as *Seamless Population Selection* design *and Sample Size Reestimation (SSR).* While both blinded and unblinded adaptations are possible, those with blinded assessment are usually less controversial and are out of scope for this chapter.

Confirmatory adaptive trials combine two main stages: a *learning stage,* which would otherwise be achieved in a phase 2 trial; and a *confirmatory stage* similar to a pivotal phase 3 trial. If prespecified, modifications of certain elements of the confirmatory stage design are allowed based on the outcome from the *learning stage* or interim analyses of the trial. At the end of the trial, data from both the stages are combined for final analysis using appropriate statistical methodology.

In this chapter, we discuss Seamless Population Selection design and Unblinded SSR for Oncology confirmatory trials. We describe the key statistical considerations and relevant methodologies. Two case studies are included to elaborate the practical application. Finally, we reflect on the key operational aspects along with current regulatory perspectives.

7.2 Seamless Population Selection Design in Oncology

Many recent cancer drugs target one or more specific biological pathways. A patient is more likely to benefit from the drug if his tumors are mediated through aberration of the specific pathway(s). Therefore, selection of the right patient population is crucial for the successful development of such targeted therapy. The traditional approaches identify the patient population in a separate phase II. Further confirmation requires a follow-up phase 3 trial. This process is time-consuming and resource intensive. A *seamless population selection design* uses a *learning stage* for population selection and a *confirmatory stage* to confirm the activity of the drug in the selected population. This approach provides benefits in terms of reduction in overall time and the number of patients necessary for the target therapy development.

The main statistical considerations for a seamless population selection design are good decision criteria for population selection after the learning stage and controlling the overall type-I error rates. Another consideration includes the correction of potential biases in the treatment effect estimates and associated confidence intervals while reporting the trial results. Finally, one needs to explore the operating characteristics of such a complex design to understand the statistical properties (e.g., type-I error, power, probability of correct selection, etc.). In this section, we provide an overview of the methods to address these statistical questions along with a case study.

7.2.1 Methods for Type-I Error Rate Control

Type-I error rate inflation in *Seamless Population Selection* design can arise due to the following:

1. Repeated testing of hypothesis: Final analysis using data from multiple stages requires testing of the same hypothesis at multiple stages. In addition, combining information from multiple trial stages is required.
2. Change in hypotheses: Testing of different sets of hypotheses at interim and final analysis.

Methodologies based on the *conditional invariance principle* [8] are powerful for combining data from multiple stages in seamless population selection trials. This methodology is flexible enough to adjust for any interim population selection decisions rule (either frequentist or Bayesian). *Combination tests* and *conditional error functions* are the most commonly used methods based on the *conditional invariance principle.* Typically, combination tests and conditional error functions are used together with *closed test procedure* [12] in seamless population selection designs.

7.2.1.1 Combination Test

Combination test along with a closed testing procedure restricts an initial set of hypotheses after each interim analysis. The overall type-I error is protected using a two-step procedure:

1. First step (closed test procedure): Separate p-values are computed at the end of each stage with adjustments based on the number of null hypotheses (e.g., number of treatment comparisons, number

of subgroups). Adjustments are based on the *closed testing principle* (Bonferroni [12], Simes 1986 [33], Hochberg and Tamhane 1987 [18], Bretz et al. 2006, 2009 [6,7]).

2. Second step (combination test): The *p*-values from each stage are combined using a combination function (e.g., the inverse Gaussian distribution).

The combination test in conjunction with closed test procedure controls the familywise type-I error rate (FWER). Examples include the Zelnorm trial (Posch et al. 2005 [29]). For further references, see Bauer and Köhne 1994 [1] and Brannath et al. 2007 [4]. A case study using the combination test approach is discussed in the next section.

7.2.1.2 Conditional Error Function

An alternative approach is the conditional error function in conjunction with the closed test principle. The conditional error function at a specific time point is the probability of rejecting the null hypothesis conditional on the data accumulated so far (Proschan and Hunsberger 1995 [30], Müller and Schäfer 2001, 2004 [27,28]). Conditional error functions in combination with closed test procedure control the FWER. Under certain conditions, both methods can be shown to be mathematically equivalent (Vandemeulebroecke 2006 [37]) and have been used in seamless confirmatory designs across the industry.

7.2.2 Statistical Tools for Interim Decision-Making

The conditional invariance principle allows for flexible interim decisions while controlling type-I error rates. Both frequentist (e.g., conditional power [CP], closed testing procedures) and Bayesian methods (e.g., predictive power) can be used for population selection. Important references in this area include Posch et al. 2005 [29], Thall 1988 [34], Schmidli et al. 2007 [31], Kimani et al. 2009 [22], and Brannath et al. 2009 [5]. For the rest of this section and case study 1, we have discussed decision rules based on *Predictive Probability of Success (PPoS)* (Brannath et al. 2009 [5]).

A popular and intuitive metric for adaptation is the *PPoS*, the conditional probability of a treatment arm or subpopulation to be statistically significant given the interim data. Together with the other relevant interim information (e.g., effect estimates, standard error), *PPoS* is often used to guide adaptations.

PPoS calculation can be frequentist or Bayesian, although the latter is more general and more powerful for complex designs. Bayesian computations use the *posterior predictive distribution* of future data. For progression-free survival (PFS) or overall survival (OS), *PPoS* calculations usually use asymptotic normality of the log-rank test statistics (Brannath et al. 2009 [5], Schoenfeld 1981 [32]). We illustrate this further in the chapter.

We define U_{ij} and I_{ij} as a log-rank test statistic and its approximate variance at analysis i for population j respectively, where $i = 1$ (end of *learning stage*), 2 (final analysis/end of the *confirmatory stage*), and $j = S$ (targeted subpopulation), or F (full population). The log-rank statistics for stage 1 and 2 can be represented as

$$\hat{\theta}_{1S} = U_{1S}/I_{1S},\ \hat{\theta}_{1S^c} = U_{1S^c}/I_{1S^c} \text{ and } \hat{\theta}_{1F} = (U_{1S} + U_{1Sc})/(I_{1S} + I_{1S^c}),$$

$$\hat{\theta}_{2S} = (U_{2S} - U_{1S})/(I_{2S} - I_{1S}),$$

$$\hat{\theta}_{2S^c} = (U_{2S^c} - U_{1S^c})/(I_{2S^c} - I_{1S^c}) \text{ and,}$$

$$\hat{\theta}_{2F} = (U_{2S} - U_{1S} + U_{2S^c} - U_{1S^c})/(I_{2F} - I_{1F})$$

where $I_{2F} = I_{2S} + I_{2S^c}$

S^c represents the non-targeted subpopulation. Using asymptotic normality of $(\hat{\theta}_{js}, \hat{\theta}_{jF} : j = 1,2)$ and conjugate non-informative priors, the posterior distribution is asymptotically Bivariate normal as follows:

$$\begin{pmatrix} \theta_S \\ \theta_F \end{pmatrix} \Bigg| \begin{pmatrix} \hat{\theta}_{1S} \\ \hat{\theta}_{1F} \end{pmatrix} \sim N_2\left(\begin{pmatrix} \hat{\theta}_{1S} \\ \hat{\theta}_{1F} \end{pmatrix}, \Sigma_1 = \begin{pmatrix} 1/I_{1S} & 1/I_{1F} \\ 1/I_{1F} & 1/I_{1F} \end{pmatrix}\right).$$

Finally, assuming $(\hat{\theta}_{1S}, \hat{\theta}_{1F})$ and $(\hat{\theta}_{2S}, \hat{\theta}_{2F})$ are independent, it follows that the predictive distribution is also Bivariate normal

$$\begin{pmatrix} \hat{\theta}_{2S} \\ \hat{\theta}_{2F} \end{pmatrix} \Bigg| \begin{pmatrix} \hat{\theta}_{1S} \\ \hat{\theta}_{1F} \end{pmatrix} \sim N_2\left(\begin{pmatrix} \hat{\theta}_{1S} \\ \hat{\theta}_{1F} \end{pmatrix}, \begin{pmatrix} 1/(I_{2S} - I_{1S}) & 1/(I_{2F} - I_{1F}) \\ 1/(I_{2F} - I_{1F}) & 1/(I_{2F} - I_{1F}) \end{pmatrix} + \Sigma_1\right).$$

Therefore, the posterior and predictive probabilities can be calculated using bivariate normal distribution. The population selection decisions at the end of the *learning stage* are as follows (Table 7.1).

Here, PPoS_F and PPoS_S are the PPoS for the full and sub-population, respectively, with P_F and P_S as decision thresholds.

TABLE 7.1

Final Analyses Hypothesis Testing Strategies

Scenario	Decision
$\text{PPOS}_F \le P_F$ and $\text{PPOS}_S \le P_S$	Stop the trial for futility
$\text{PPOS}_F \le P_F$ and $\text{PPOS}_S > P_S$	Continue with the targeted subpopulation
$\text{PPOS}_F > P_F$ and $\text{PPOS}_S \le P_S$	Continue with full population
$\text{PPOS}_F > P_F$ and $\text{PPOS}_S > P_S$ but the effect is driven by the targeted subpopulation	Continue with the targeted subpopulation
$\text{PPOS}_F > P_F$, $\text{PPOS}_S \ge P_S$ and both targeted and non-targeted subpopulations are promising	Continue with full population

7.2.3 Correcting Bias for Treatment Effect Estimates

Another concern in seamless population selection designs is the potential bias associated with estimates of treatment effects and associated confidence intervals (Hung et al. 2011, 2014 [19,20]). Since interim adaptations often select groups with promising estimates, there is the potential to overestimate treatment effects. On the other hand, if interim treatment effects are small, the trial recruitment may be stopped, which may result in underestimation.

The bias topic continues to be controversial (Bauer et al. 2010 [2]). In general, bias-corrected methods are not routinely used in clinical trials and the uncorrected point estimates and confidence intervals are usually reported. The most commonly used methods include one-sided repeated confidence intervals based on the p-clud condition (Brannath et al. 2009 [5]), removal of bias (Bowden and Glimm 2008 [3]), and bias corrections (Carreras and Brannath 2013 [9], Posch et al. 2005 [29]). Fortunately, for confirmatory studies with large sample sizes, biases for standard (non-adjusted) treatment effect estimates are generally negligible.

Nevertheless, it is important to understand the potential concerns and be prepared to address them. Sensitivity analyses with different methods can be used to assess the impact of adaptation on final treatment effect estimates. To assess a potential drift in patient populations, pre and post adaptation, exploratory analyses for pre- and post-adaptation estimates should be envisaged as appropriate.

Finally, adequate considerations must be given at the design stage to assess the frequentist operating characteristics. Most important ones include type-I error, power, and probability of correct decision at the interim analysis. Closed form expressions for these metrics are generally not available. Therefore, simulations play an important role in assessing the operating characteristics under different scenarios.

7.2.4 Case Study 1

In this section, we illustrate a hypothetical seamless population selection design in oncology. The goal of this design is to select and confirm a biomarker-based patient population for an experimental drug (Treatment A) in a specific tumor type. Three hundred and eighty-nine patients with a specific tumor type and a known biomarker status (activated or nonactivated) are to be randomized equally either to Treatment A or control (C). The design has two stages—*learning* and *confirmatory*. The objective of the *learning* stage is to select a population (full population or biomarker-activated subpopulation) for the *confirmatory* stage. The confirmatory stage is used to confirm the efficacy of Treatment A in the selected population. For both stages of the trial, the primary objective of the trial is to compare Treatment A with C in terms of PFS. Stopping the study early for the lack of efficacy (futility)

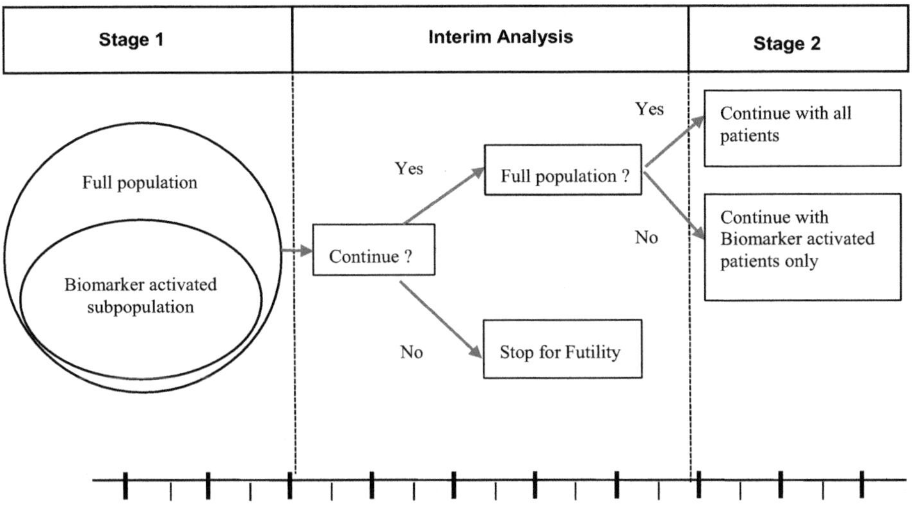

FIGURE 7.1
Study design for seamless confirmatory study with adaptive population selection.

will be considered if neither the full nor the biomarker-activated subpopulation looks promising at the end of the *learning* stage. There is no plan to stop the study at the interim analysis for efficacy (Figure 7.1).

7.2.4.1 Statistical Hypothesis Testing Strategy

Assuming a proportional hazard model for PFS within the full population and the biomarker-activated subpopulation, the following two null hypotheses will be tested at the end of the trial:

i. Full population: H_{0F}: $\theta_1 \geq 0$ vs. H_{1F}: $\theta_1 < 0$
ii. Biomarker-activated subpopulation: H_{0S}: $\theta_2 \geq 0$ vs. H_{1S}: $\theta_2 < 0$

Here θ_1 and θ_2 are the log hazard ratio (HR) of PFS (Treatment A vs C) in the full population and the biomarker-activated subpopulation, respectively. The primary analysis of PFS is performed at the end of the confirmatory stage using log-rank tests. For the full population, the log-rank test is stratified by the biomarker-activated status.

Data from the learning and confirmatory stages are combined for the final analysis. A combination test procedure is used to maintain the FWER at 2.5%. The methodology for this trial is adapted from Brannath et al. 2009 [5]. A weighted inverse normal combination function is used for testing H_{0F} and H_{0S} in a stepwise fashion under a closed testing framework.

- **Step 1 (Hypotheses for multiple populations):** Since two hypotheses are initially of interest, a closed testing principle is used separately at each phase to maintain the FWER at level 2.5% one-sided. The test for the global null hypothesis ($H_{0F} \cap H_{0S}$) is based on the Hochberg-adjusted p-value.
- **Step 2 (Combining data from different stages):** All p-values from the learning and confirmatory phase for individual and intersection hypotheses will be combined using inverse normal combination function (with weights w_1 and w_2):

$$C(p_1, p_2) = w_1\Phi^{-1}(1-p_1) + w_2\Phi^{-1}(1-p_2) \text{ with } w_1{}^2 + w_2{}^2 = 1$$

Φ denotes the cumulative distribution function of the standard normal distribution. Prespecified fixed weights based on the proportion of events at each stage are used. This means that the weights are $w_1 = 0.63$ and $w_2 = 0.77$. The hypothesis testing strategy is detailed in Table 7.2.

Here, p_{1F}, p_{1S}, p_{2F}, and p_{2S} are nominal log-rank p-values for the *learning* and *confirmatory* phases for the individual hypotheses of the full and biomarker-active subpopulation. Furthermore, q_1 and q_2 are the Hochberg-adjusted p-values for the intersection hypothesis (qi = min{2min(piS, piF), max(piS, piF)}; $i = 1,2$). Note that, if only biomarker-activated subpopulation is selected at the end of the *learning phase,* in the final testing, Hochberg's procedure is required for the *learning phase* data but not for the *confirmatory phase* data. Therefore, the combination function in Table 7.2 only involves q_1. Otherwise, if the full population is carried forward after the *learning stage,* Hochberg's procedure is required for both *learning* and *confirmatory phases.* Therefore, the combination function for the final testing involves both q_1 and q_2. For further details, see Brannath et al. 2009 [5].

7.2.4.2 Interim Analysis

The interim population selection is based on *PPoS*. Either the full population or the biomarker-active subpopulation will be selected based on sufficiently high predictive probabilities that the respective populations will succeed

TABLE 7.2

Final Analyses Hypothesis Testing Strategies

Population Selected at the End of *Learning* Phase	Hypothesis Testing Strategy
Continue with the biomarker subpopulation only	Reject H_{0S} if $C(q_1, p_{2s}) \geq 1.96$ and $C(p_{1s}, p_{2s}) \geq 1.96$
Population selected at the end of the *learning* phase.	Hypothesis testing strategy.
Continue with the full population	Reject H_{0F} if $C(q_1, q_2) \geq 1.96$ and $C(p_{1F}, p_{2F}) \geq 1.96$ Reject H_{0S} if $C(q_1, q_2) \geq 1.96$ and $C(p_{1S}, p_{2S}) \geq 1.96$

(achieve statistical significance) at the end. For this design, the *PPoS* decision thresholds for full and biomarker-activated subpopulation (P_F and P_S in Section 7.2) are set to 45% and 35%.

To continue the trial with full population at the *confirmatory stage,* it is important to ensure that Treatment A has activity in the biomarker-nonactivated subpopulation also. In addition to the *PPoS* criteria, the activity of Treatment A is evaluated using posterior probability. A posterior probability of at least 70% confirms the preliminary efficacy of Treatment A in the nonactivated subpopulation. All thresholds are confirmed via simulation. The trial is stopped for futility if PPoS is low for both full and biomarker-active populations.

7.2.4.3 Sample Size

The sample size calculation is based on the log-rank test and the following assumptions:

a. Biomarker prevalence rate: 45%
b. Enrollment rate: 30 patients per month
c. Placebo median for PFS for full and biomarker-activated subpopulation: 7 months
d. Alternative hypothesis: a 42% risk reduction in PFS (HR = 0.58) by Treatment A for full or biomarker-activated subpopulation. This corresponds to at least a 5-month increase in median PFS for Treatment A over placebo.
e. Lost to follow-up rate: 15%

Given the abovementioned assumptions and one-sided $\alpha = 2.5\%$, an initial sample is performed using EAST 6.4 [13]. The final sample size is based on the computer simulations under different scenarios. It ensures approximately 90% power when the alternative hypothesis is true for both the full and biomarker-activated subpopulation. The timing of interim analysis or end of the *learning* stage ensures a high probability for correct population selection. The final sample size for the two stages is provided as follows.

a. The *learning* stage ends after 84 PFS events in the full population. At this time, the expected number of events in the biomarker-activated subpopulation is 40–55.
b. If the full population is selected at the end of the *learning* stage, approximately 210 PFS events are required for the final analysis.
c. If the biomarker subpopulation is selected at the end of the *learning* stage, approximately 176 PFS events are required for the final analysis.

TABLE 7.3

Type-I and Power Calculation via Simulation

Underlying Treatment Effect HR			Probability to Decision at the End of Learning Stage		
Biomarker-Activated Patients (S)	Biomarker Nonactivated Patients (S^C)	Overall Trial Power	Continue With Full Population (*F*)	Continue with Biomarker-Activated Subpopulation Only (*S*)	Futility
1	1	1.8%	13.3%	9.9%	76.8%
0.58	1	67.6%	33.1%	46.1%	20.8%
0.58	0.58	89.4%	88.4%	4.5%	7.0%

7.2.4.4 Design Operating Characteristics

Simulations are carried out to explore the impact of the interim analyses and the adaptive design features on the power of the study and to optimize the sample size considerations. The simulations take into account all possible trial decision scenarios. The operating characteristics are provided in Table 7.3. Under the null scenario, the proposed design demonstrates strong control of the type-1 error at 0.025. The power to reject at least one null hypothesis when Treatment A is active in both biomarker-activated subpopulation and the full population is above 89%. Moreover, the population selection decisions are reasonable under different scenarios.

Further simulations are conducted to understand the impact of the enrolment rate and prevalence of the biomarker subpopulation. They play an important role in understanding the overall sample size and duration of the trial, which has a significant impact on the operational and commercial aspects.

7.3 Sample Size Reestimation in Oncology

In this section, we discuss an unblinded SSR design. This design allows for on-trial modification of the trial sample size based on unblinded interim results or other factors such as external information. The adjusted sample size ensures a desired power of the design when the assumed treatment effect at the design stage requires modification (Chen et. al. 2004 [11], Tsiatis and Mehta 2003 [35]). As a general rule, it is recommended to only consider adaptive methods for sample size increase [36]. There are two critical statistical considerations while contemplating an unblinded SSR design:

1. Interim decision for trial sample size readjustment, and
2. Maintaining the overall type-I error rate below the specified α-level.

7.3.1 Decision Rule for Sample Size Reassessment

Similar to the other adaptive designs, an SSR design has two stages. Assessment of sample size increment takes place after the end of stage 1. A good decision rule for the sample size increment depends upon the likelihood of the trial success contingent on the current sample size and the observed treatment effect estimate at stage 1. There are three possible outcomes at the end of stage 1:

1. *No change in sample size*: If the observed evidence at the interim is comparable or more favorable compared to the original assumptions.
2. *Increase in sample size*: If the interim estimates indicate that the treatment benefit is less optimistic yet clinically meaningful and therefore a trial with increased sample size is likely to be successful.
3. *Stop for futility*: If treatment benefit seems unsatisfactory.

Metrics used for interim decision in population selection design are applicable for unblinded SSR designs. Following Posch et al. 2005 [29], we discuss the use of CP. The CP is the probability of success of a trial given the stage 1 data and assuming a specific true treatment effect. Often, it is calculated for different assumptions about the true effect size (e.g., effect under the null, effect under the originally assumed alternative, or observed effect estimate treated as if it were the true effect). A *promising zone* can be defined as a range of CP values (CP_{min}, CP_{max}) for which a moderate sample size increase would achieve a desired overall power (Müller and Schäfer 2001 [27]). However, reassessement of the sample size based on stage 1 data carries a risk of unintentional unblinding of the trial in certain situations. For example, CP is a function of the number of events and observed HR at stage 1 in time-to-event trials. Therefore, one can approximately calculate the HR from stage 1, given the CP boundaries and increase in the number of events. In order to prevent this, a flat increase in sample size is typically planned for any value of CP in the promising zone. For example, if $0.20 \leq CP < 0.8$, the overall sample is increased by 50%. This prevents the back-calculation of the treatment effect based on interim result. For any SSR rule, it is important to not only take into account its operating efficiency but also its operating risks and complexity in terms of its implementation.

7.3.2 Type-I Error Control

It is important to emphasize that the number of observations available at the end of an adaptive trial with SSR is a random variable. Hence, testing at the final analysis while ignoring that the sample size was not fixed in advance often leads to a biased inference. Combination tests are commonly used to control type-I error rates in adaptive designs with SSR.

7.3.2.1 Combination Tests

As stated in Section 7.2.1, we have described the combination test as a method for combining *p*-values from different stages of a trial. Cui, Hung, and Wang, 1999 (CHW) [10] have proposed to use predefined weights for combining test statistics from different stages in unblinded SSR. The proposed method protects the type-I error. However, it is less efficient as the weighting of the stagewise test statistics is not proportional to the sample size at each stage. Müller and Schäfer (2001) [24] and Gao et al. 2008 [15] have proposed an adjusted test statistic, by combining the interim result with the final trial result in group sequential fashion. In the next section, we have illustrated the practical utility of CHW using a case study.

Other notable work in this area includes Gao et al. 2008 [15] and Mehta & Pocock 2011 [24]. The authors showed that if the lower bound of the *promising zone* is at least 50%, the unadjusted Wald statistic can replace the weighted CHW statistic to control the type-I error rate. Mehta & Pocock 2011[23] have also recommended that the sample size adjustment is more beneficial only if interim analysis results are within the promising zone. However, criticisms of this approach include the loss of power and the decision rule based on CP using an unstable point estimate at interim (Glimm 2011 [17]). Mehta & Pocock 2011 [25] have also shown that the power loss is negligible in general.

Similar to the *seamless population selection* design, simulations play an important role in unblinded SSR. Simulation studies are necessary to evaluate the frequentist operating characteristics of an SSR design under a wide number of scenarios. The utility of simulation methods are elaborated in Case study 2.

7.3.3 Case Study 2

In this example, we present a case study to illustrate the use of unblinded SSR in a confirmatory oncology clinical trial with OS as the primary endpoint. Consider an experimental drug (Treatment A) being administered in combination with a standard of care (Treatment B). A double-blind placebo-controlled study is to investigate the survival advantage of the combination over the standard of care plus placebo. Although the trial is designed with the final analysis after 305 deaths, there are uncertainties about the effect of Treatment A in the studied indication. A reliable assumption about the magnitude of the target treatment effect (HR) is difficult prior to the trial. Therefore, additional flexibility is required to mitigate this uncertainty.

Two interim analyses are planned approximately at 40% and 70% information to evaluate the initial design assumptions. In one of the two interims, an unblinded SSR is planned. Furthermore, the design also has the provision to stop at interim for overwhelming efficacy or futility. Stopping at interim for futility or efficacy is guided by the O'Brien Fleming beta and alpha-spending functions, respectively. For example, if an unblinded SSR is performed at the

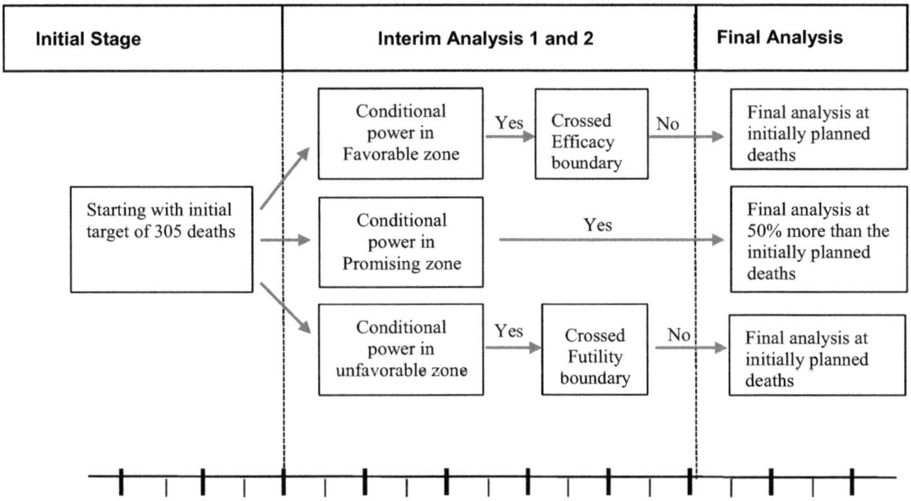

FIGURE 7.2
Study design with unblinded SSR.

first interim, the main purpose of the second interim is stopping for efficacy. No further SSR will take place at the second interim in such a case (Figure 7.2).

The initial sample size is calculated using a three-look group sequential design, with the possibility of stopping for futility or efficacy at each interim. The trial is initially powered at 80% for an alternative hypothesis HR = 0.72 requiring 305 events. An HR of 0.78 would still be clinically meaningful. To design a trial with 80% power for this alternative hypothesis requires 533 events. However, with current uncertainty about the efficacy of the experimental treatment, committing to such a larger study would be cost and resource prohibitive. As an alternative, an unblinded SSR is considered. This design allows the trial to start using the original assumptions (HR = 0.72). However, there is an option for increasing the final sample size based on the interim analyses results.

7.3.3.1 Decision for Sample Size Reestimation

In this design, the sample size increase can occur either at interim analysis 1 or interim analysis 2. The unblinded SSR will be based on CP and promising zone based on clinical consideration. The decision boundaries at interim analyses are as follows:

I. SSR at Interim Analysis 1:

a. **Favorable**: If CP under current estimate ≥0.8 (or equivalently observed HR ≤ 0.74) and does not cross the efficacy boundary, keep the total target sample size at 305 deaths and perform the next interim at 0.7*305 deaths as originally planned.

b. **Promising**: If 0.23 ≤ CP under current estimate < 0.8 (or equivalently observed 0.74 ≤ HR ≤ 0.85), continue and increase the number of finally targeted events by 50% of originally planned. The next interim analysis and final analysis will be performed after 321 deaths (0.7*1.5*305) and 458 (1.5*305) deaths, respectively.

c. **Unfavorable**: If CP under current estimate <0.23 (or equivalently observed HR > 0.85) and does not cross futility boundary, keep the total target sample size at 305 deaths and perform the next interim at 214 (0.7*305) deaths as originally planned.

II. SSR Interim Analysis 2:

If SSR is performed in the interim analysis 1, the goal of the interim analysis 2 is early efficacy assessment. No additional SSR will be done. Otherwise, an unblinded SSR will be decided as follows:

a. **Favorable**: If CP under current estimate ≥ 0.8 (or equivalently observed HR ≤ 0.76) and does not cross efficacy boundary, continue to 305 deaths.

b. **Promising**: If 0.15 ≤ CP under current estimate < 0.8 (or equivalently observed 0.76 ≤ HR < 0.85), continue and increase the total number of events to 50% of originally planned. The final analysis will be performed after 458 (1.5*305) deaths.

c. **Unfavorable**: If CP under current estimate < 0.15 (or equivalently observed HR > 0.85) and does not cross futility boundary, continue to 305 deaths.

The decision boundaries are based on the upper bound for statistical significance under alternative hypothesis HR = 0.78, and ensuring adequate control of type-1 error. If sample size is increased after interim analysis 1, the timing of interim analysis 2 and final analysis needs to be adjusted in order to maintain 70% and 100% information fractions, respectively. On the basis of CHW 1999 [10], it ensures the invariance of variance–covariance of the interim test statistic. Therefore, no change is required for interim efficacy and futility boundary.

7.3.3.2 Statistical Hypothesis Testing Strategy

The interim and final analysis will be based on a log-rank test. The hypothesis testing within *promising zones* is based on the re-weighted test statistics (CHW 1999) [10]. The reweighted test is based on a linear combination of the test statistics from three stages. The weights reflect the planned number of events at the stage from the original design. The final test statistic is:

$$Z^{*}_{CHW} = \sqrt{\frac{n_{Interim1}}{n_{Final}}} Z_{Stage1} + \sqrt{\frac{n_{Final} - n_{Interim1}}{n_{Final}}} Z_{Stage2}$$

Z_{Stage1} and Z_{Stage2} are stagewise log-rank statistics by assuming an independent increment. For additional methods for combining data from multiple stages in time-to-event trials, see Irle and Schäfer 2012 [21] and Magirr et al. 2014 [23]. $\boldsymbol{Z}^{*}_{CHW} > 1.96$ results trial success.

7.3.3.3 Design Operating Characteristics

Table 7.4 displays the unconditional power and expected number of events of the proposed design. The overall type-I error is well protected under the proposed SSR scheme. Compared to the fixed sample design, there is a 5% gain in power when underlying HR = 0.78. However, the unconditional power is not useful to understand the full benefit of SSR. One also needs to look into CP (Mehta and Pocock 2011 [24]). The expected study duration in Table 7.4 is calculated by assuming that the enrolment rate remains the same from the beginning of the study.

In order to understand the design further, Table 7.5 displays the operating characteristics conditional on the zone into which the CP falls at the first and second interim analyses. The table reveals a substantial gain in power as compared to the original design if the interim outcome falls in the *promising zone*, due to the increase in the sample size. If the interim outcome falls in the favorable zone, the design shows a good power without any increase in size. The increase in power in the promising zone is similar when the SSR is done at interim 1 or 2; however, there is a substantial increase in the study duration if the SSR is done at the later interim. Finally, the design shows low power and no increase in the sample size if the interim outcome falls in the unfavorable zone.

To summarize, the proposed unblinded SSR design provides the opportunity to increase the sample size only when the results of the interim analyses fall in the *promising zone*. However, the choice of the SSR strategy also needs to

TABLE 7.4

Type-I Error and Power for the Sample Size Reestimation of 50% at Interim Analyses 1 or 2

	IA1			IA2		
	Overall Power	**Expected Study Duration**	**Expected # of Events**	**Overall Power**	**Expected Study Duration**	**Expected # of Events**
HR = 1	2.49	35	213	2.38	34	211
HR = 0.78	61	52	295	61	53	299
HR = 0.72	84	50	280	85	53	292

TABLE 7.5

Operating Characteristics of SSR Designs Conditional on First and Second Interim Outcome Under HR = 0.78 and HR = 0.72

		Interim Analysis 1				Interim Analysis 2			
True HR	**Zone**	**Probability[a] (%)**	**Power**	**Study Duration**	**# of Events[c]**	**Probability[a] (%)**	**Power**	**Study Duration**	**# of Events[c]**
HR = 0.78	Futility	10	0	25	122	10	0	25	122
	Unfavorable	26	34	52	301	26	17	52	305
	Promising Zone								
	Original Design	27	59	50	290	24	58	52	305
	CHW method		79	72	411		82	81	458
	Favorable[b]	37	84	44	254	39	94	43	244
HR = 0.72	Futility	4	0	25	122	4	0	25	122
	Unfavorable	14	54	52	299	8	21	53	305
	Promising Zone								
	Original Design	28	80	49	277	25	74	53	305
	Promising Zone		93	69	380		91	84	458
	Favorable[b]	54	94	43	239	63	97	42	235

[a] Probability of being in a zone.
[b] Interim Analysis 2: Efficacy Stopping included in the Favorable zone.
[c] Expected # of events.

be evaluated in terms of the practical feasibility. The timing of SSR is critical. An early SSR decision will be based on an immature estimate of HR. However, a late SSR may render the possibility of additional enrolment infeasible.

7.4 Operational Considerations of Adaptive Design for Confirmatory Trials

Adaptive trials are more complex to implement than conventional trials and their successful implementation requires careful consideration of the operational aspects. For confirmatory trials, it is critical to ensure that the unblinded interim results do not influence the ongoing study conduct and monitoring of patients. Due to the unblinding of interim data and the resulting design adaptations in confirmatory adaptive trials, operational biases may raise questions about the integrity of study conduct. Since operational biases cannot be quantified, adequate processes to prevent them must be in place.

Two important operational aspects of adaptive confirmatory trial design are proper documentation and an independent data monitoring committee (DMC). The study protocol must contain the key design aspects (e.g., sample size, adaptation decision, and methods for type-I error control). In addition, the statistical methods for testing and estimation need to be clearly specified in a statistical analysis plan. The health authorities often ask for simulation programs and results for review. Therefore, user-friendly documentation of simulation programs is helpful.

DMCs play an important role in adaptive design. It is therefore crucial to select DMC members with the right expertise and experience. For unblinded data analysis and presentation to the DMC, an independent statistical organization must be engaged. A well-documented and clearly written DMC charter explaining the role of DMC members, sponsor plan, and communication plan must be in place.

Other aspects include handling of randomization, drug supply, efficient data capturing & management plan, biomarker assay validation and availability plans. Cross-functional collaboration is crucial to ensure an efficient trial conduct.

7.5 Regulatory Guidance on Adaptive Designs for Confirmatory Trials

The FDA and the EMA have both released guidance discussing their view on the operational and statistical aspects for adaptive designs. The following shows how FDA and EMA guidance have evolved over time:

- In 2007, the EMA issued its "Reflection Paper on Methodological Issues in Confirmatory Clinical Trials Planned with an Adaptive Design" [14]. The paper does not discuss any specific statistical methods. However, while it recognizes the value of flexible designs in early drug development, it expresses concerns about too much flexibility in confirmatory trials.
- In 2010, the FDA's Center for Drug Evaluation and Research and the Center for Biologics Evaluation and Research issued a joint draft guidance for adaptive designs, which emphasizes *adequate and well-controlled* phase 3 trials [36]. This guidance, as well as other reports, encourages sponsors to use innovative designs. Designs are classified into: 1) designs whose properties are *well-understood*, such as group sequential designs or designs using blinded sample size reassessments; and 2) more innovative or *less well-understood* designs, for which experience is still sparse. For the latter, which includes the adaptive confirmatory designs, sponsors are urged to seek early discussion with the FDA. A revised guideline is released on September 2018.

Sponsors of clinical trials need to seek health authority feedback on adaptive designs early in the planning phase. Some important points for discussion include adaptation rules and blinding procedures (Gaydos et al. 2009 [16]). When submitting a seamless confirmatory design for regulatory review, detailed information must be available in the briefing package, protocol, statistical analysis plan, simulation report, and DMC charter.

7.6 Discussion

Confirmatory clinical trials are a critical component in a drug development program. A positive outcome at this stage directly impacts the market authorization approval, and therefore access to novel therapies for patients. Confirmatory trials carry inherent risks and uncertainty and thus require strategies to mitigate risks. Unblinded *sample size reestimation* and *seamless population selection* designs provide opportunities to mitigate risk via trial adaptations.

Adaptive confirmatory trials are not appropriate for all situations. They pose operational and statistical challenges, which may question the validity of study conduct and study results if not carefully planned. The operational challenges include drug supply, changes in randomization, and improper dissemination of interim decisions. Regarding statistical challenges, strict control of type-I error rates is essential for registration. These challenges can be overcome by appropriate planning and procedures. Therefore, upfront investment of time and resources is critical. These investments must be weighed against the potential benefits of a seamless confirmatory trial.

Acknowledgments

We would like to thank Beat Neuenschwander, Venkata Sasikiran Goteti, Bharani Dharan, Eulodge Kpamegan, and David Mills for their contributions, as well as Michael Branson and Ekkehard Glimm for valuable discussions, inputs, and support.

References

1. Bauer P and Köhne K (1994). Evaluation of experiments with adaptive interim analyses. *Biometrics*, 50, 1029–1041.
2. Bauer P, Köhne F, Brannath W and Posch M (2010). Selection and bias - two hostile brothers. *Statistics in Medicine*, 29, 1–13.
3. Bowden J and Glimm E (2008). Unbiased estimation of selected treatment means in two-stage trials. *Biometrical Journal*, 50(4), 515–527.
4. Brannath W, Koenig F and Bauer P (2007). Multiplicity and flexibility in clinical trials. *Pharmaceutical Statistics*, 6(3), 205–216.
5. Brannath W, Zuber E, Branson M, Bretz F, Gallo P, Posch M and Racine-Poon A (2009). Confirmatory adaptive designs with Bayesian decision tools for a targeted therapy in oncology. *Statistics in Medicine*, 28(10), 1445–1463.
6. Bretz F, Schmidli H, Koenig F, Racine A and Maurer W (2006). Confirmatory seamless phase II/III clinical trials with hypotheses selection at interim: General concepts (with discussion). *Biometrical Journal*, 48(4), 623–634.
7. Bretz F, Maurer W, Brannath W and Posch M (2009). A graphical approach to sequentially rejective multiple test procedures. *Statistics in Medicine*, 28(4), 586–604.
8. Bretz F, Koenig F, Brannath W, Glimm E and Posch M (2009). Adaptive designs for confirmatory clinical trials. *Statistics in Medicine*, 28(8), 1181–1217.
9. Carreras M and Brannath W (2013). Shrinkage estimation in two-stage adaptive designs with midtrial treatment selection. *Statistics in medicine*, 32(10), 1677–1690.
10. Cui L, Hung HMJ and Wang SJ (1999). Modification of sample size in group sequential clinical trials. *Biometrics*, 55, 853–857.
11. Chen, YH, DeMets, DL and Lan, KK (2004). Increasing the sample size when the unblinded interim result is promising. *Statistics in Medicine*, 23, 1023–1038.
12. Dmitrienko A, Tamhane AC and Bretz F (Editors) (2009). *Multiple Testing Problems in Pharmaceutical Statistics*. Chapmann & Hall/CRC. Biostatistics Series.
13. EAST 6.4 Software: Cytel Corporation.
14. European Medicine Agency (2007). Reflection Paper on Methodological Issues in Confirmatory Clinical Trials Planned with an Adaptive Design. http://www.ema.europa.eu/docs/en_GB/document_library/Scientific_guideline/2009/09/WC500003616.pdf.
15. Gao P, Ware, JH and Mehta CR (2008). Sample size re-estimation for adaptive sequential design in clinical trials. *Journal of Biopharmaceutical Statistic*, 18, 1184–1196.

16. Gaydos B, Anderson KM, Berry D, Burnham N, Chuang-Stein CJ, Dubinak J, Fardipour P, Gallo P, Givens S, Lewis R, Maca J, Pinheiro J, Pritchett Y and Krams M (2009). Good practices for adaptive clinical trials in pharmaceutical product development. *Drug Informational Journal*, 43, 539–556.
17. Glimm E (2011). Comments on 'Adaptive increase in sample size when interim results are promising: A practical guide with examples' by C. R. Mehta and S. J. Pocock. *Statistics in Medicine*, 31(1), 98–99.
18. Hochberg Y and Tamhane AC (1987). Multiple comparison procedures. *Biometrika*, 73, 751–754.
19. Hung HMJ, Wang SJ and O'Neill R (2011). Flexible design clinical trial methodology in regulatory applications. *Statistics in Medicine*, 30, 1519–1527.
20. Hung HMJ, Wang SJ and Yanga P (2014). Some challenges with statistical inference in adaptive designs. *Journal of Biopharmaceutical Statistics*, 24(5), 1059–1072.
21. Irle, S and Shafer, H (2012). Interim design modifications in time to-event studies. *Journal of the American Statistical Association*, 107, 341–348.
22. Kimani PK, Stallard N and Hutton JL (2009). Dose selection in seamless phase II/III clinical trials based on efficacy and safety. *Statistics in Medicine*, 28, 917–936.
23. Magirr, D, Jaki T, Koening F and Posch M (2014). Adaptive survival trials. Technical report, Section of Medical Statistics, Medical University of Vienna, Vienna, Austria.
24. Mehta CR and Pocock SJ (2011). Adaptive increase in sample size when interim results are promising: A practical guide with examples. *Statistics in Medicine*, 30, 3267–3284.
25. Mehta CR and Pocock SJ (2011). Comments on "Adaptive increase in sample size when interim results are promising: A practical guide with examples" by C. R. Mehta and S. J. Pocock: Authors reply. *Statistics in Medicine*, 31(1), 99–100.
26. Miller E, Gallo P, IIe W, Kammerman LA, Koury K, Maca J, Jiang Q, Walton MK, Wang C, Woo K, Fuller C and Jemiai Y (2017). DIA's adaptive design scientific working group (ADSWG): Best practices case studies for "less well-understood" adaptive designs. *Therapeutic Innovation & Regulatory Science*, 51(1), 77–88.
27. Müller HH and Schäfer H (2001). Adaptive group sequential designs for clinical trials: combining the advantages of adaptive and of classical group sequential approaches. *Biometrics*, 57, 886–891.
28. Müller HH and Schäfer H (2004). A general statistical principle for changing a design any time during the course of a trial. *Statistics in Medicine*, 23, 2497–2508.
29. Posch M, Koenig F, Branson M, Brannath W, Dunger-Baldauf C and Bauer P (2005). Testing and estimation in flexible group sequential designs with adaptive treatment selection. *Statistics in Medicine*, 24(24), 3697–3714.
30. Proschan MA and Hunsberger SA (1995). Designed extension of studies based on conditional power, Biometrics. *Biometrics*, 51, 1315–1324.
31. Schmidli H, Bretz F and Racine-Poon A (2007). Bayesian predictive power for interim adaptation in seamless phase II/III trials where the endpoint is survival up to some specified time point. *Statistics in Medicine*, 26, 4925–4938.
32. Schoenfeld D (1981). The asymptotic properties of nonparametric tests for comparing survival distributions. *Biometrika*, 68, 316–319.
33. Simes RJ (1986). An improved Bonferroni procedure for multiple tests of significance. *Biometrika*, 73, 751–754.

34. Thall PF, Simon R and Ellenberg SS (1988). Two-stage selection and testing designs for comparative clinical trials. *Biometrika*, 75, 303–310.
35. Tsiatis, AA and Mehta, C (2003). On the inefficiency of the adaptive design for monitoring clinical trials. *Biometrika*, 20, 367–378.
36. US Department of Health and Human Services (2010). Food and Drug Administration. Guidance for Industry: Adaptive Design Clinical Trials for Drugs and Biologics Draft Guidance. http://www.fda.gov/downloads/drugs/guidancecomplianceregulatoryinformation/guidances/ucm201790.pdf.
37. Vandemeulebroecke M (2006). An investigation of two-stage tests. *Statistica Sinica*, 16, 933–951.

8

Safety Monitoring and Analysis in Oncology Trials

Anastasia Ivanova
University of North Carolina at Chapel Hill

Qi Jiang
Seattle Genetics

Olga Marchenko
Bayer Pharmaceutical

Richard C. Zink
TARGET PharmaSolutions
University of North Carolina at Chapel Hill

CONTENTS

8.1 Introduction: Safety Challenges

The safety assessment of any new drug is critical and there are a number of references on the topic (Jiang and Xia 2014; Snapinn and Jiang 2016). Benefits of the treatment must outweigh its risks to ensure a positive benefit–risk (BR) profile and there has been an increased emphasis on early and critical safety evaluation to ensure patient safety throughout the drug life cycle. There are some unique aspects in the assessment of safety for cancer treatments. One such difference is that patients are more willing to accept a greater degree of toxicity in order to obtain an important benefit than they would be for less grievous conditions. In addition, phase I clinical trials for cancer treatments are typically performed on the patients for which the treatment is intended, making it important to proactively plan for comprehensive safety evaluation and signal detection at the start of the development program. Statisticians should be intimately involved in this process and contribute their expertise to safety data collection and analysis, reporting, and data visualization.

Statistical methodologies for analyzing patient safety are less comprehensive than they are for efficacy outcomes. Methods are generally descriptive in nature due to the following challenges:

- Studies are often underpowered to detect treatment differences for safety endpoints;
- There are numerous safety endpoints to consider, including adverse events (AEs), laboratory measurements, and electrocardiograms (ECG). Without proper multiplicity adjustment, this may result in potential false-positive findings. On the other hand, strict adherence for multiple comparisons can leave little power to detect signals;
- Safety outcomes have important characteristics to consider including duration, severity, and investigator's assessment of causal relationship to drug, resulting in numerous sensitivity analyses;
- Safety events may occur spontaneously at any time during the trial, and may include events that are not expected to occur for the disease under investigation;
- Medical classifications may be inaccurate;
- BR assessments are challenging and the methodologies are currently evolving.

In this chapter, we discuss the challenges related to safety evaluation and share our thoughts on how to apply statistical thinking and methodologies to enhance the collection, analysis, reporting, and interpretation of safety data. The remainder of this chapter is organized as follows: Section 8.2 describes the program-wide safety analysis plan and the statistical analysis plan for the integrated summary of safety, documents which summarize the safety analyses to be conducted for the entire clinical development program, and outline the responsibilities of the data monitoring committee; Section 8.3 discusses AE monitoring, highlighting differences in approach between phase II and III; Section 8.4 provides an overview of safety reporting, including subgroup analysis and meta-analysis; Section 8.5 provides a brief conclusion.

8.2 Planning Safety Monitoring and Analyses

8.2.1 Analysis Plans

Safety evaluation is critical for drug development. To ensure systematic safety monitoring and evaluation, one needs a proactive safety evaluation that can be performed objectively and in a timely manner. Having the necessary safety-related documents, such as a risk management plan (RMP), can facilitate safety evaluation. However, the RMP does not consider any of the statistical aspects of development activities, so it must be complemented by a more focused document called a program-wide safety analysis plan (PSAP). The PSAP often contains the following sections: background, general plan, data generation, fata structure and content, methods for analysis, presentation and reporting, and problem-oriented summary for AEs of special interest (AESIs). A PSAP has been recommended by the Safety Planning, Evaluation and Reporting Team (Crowe et al. 2009), but it is currently not required by regulatory agencies. Nevertheless, several sponsors have adopted and implemented a PSAP (or a similar document by a different name) for documenting the appropriate data to be collected and the analyses to be performed in order to characterize the safety profile of the new therapy throughout the development life cycle. As added benefits, the PSAP can facilitate ongoing interactions with regulatory agencies regarding current safety strategies and can aid in the evaluation of the BR profile of the new therapy in the post-marketing stage.

The PSAP may be considered redundant with the statistical analysis plan for the integrated summary of safety (iSAP), but, in fact, these two documents can be very different. The PSAP provides a systematic way to evaluate safety at a product level and contains plans for both prospective and retrospective safety analyses. The contents of a PSAP are flexible and can be amended as needed throughout the product life cycle. With respect to timing, development of the PSAP can be done as early as during phase II product development, with input from different functional groups such as biostatistics, safety, clinical, and regulatory. The iSAP, on the other hand, is generally finalized quite late in the drug development process, often while phase III studies are being conducted, though prior to the unblinding of any these trials. Further, the iSAP has a more limited scope, only covering the period up to the drug submission.

8.2.2 Data Monitoring Committees

A data monitoring committee (DMC) is established primarily to protect the well-being of the trial participants through periodic review of safety outcomes for an ongoing trial. Should a safety signal appear, these reviews may result in recommendations to the sponsor regarding modifications to the study, including dropping treatment arms with higher and potentially more toxic doses, dropping arms with lower and potentially ineffective doses, or stopping the study outright. With the increased use of adaptive designs, some unique features of the DMC may need to be modified when the protocol contains adaptive elements; these features include the composition and functioning of the DMC. Although we focus on pharmaceutical industry–sponsored trials, much of this discussion can be applied to other trials as well.

In general, a fully independent DMC is needed for a phase III study to ensure the safety of trial participants and to protect the integrity of the study. A few factors that influence the need for a DMC include the seriousness of the medical condition and the level of knowledge about the investigational agent. Primary responsibilities for a DMC are to monitor the safety outcomes of the trial participants, and, increasingly, to review efficacy data in order to evaluate trade-offs in the BR profile. A study can have boundaries for stopping for efficacy, stopping for futility, and stopping for safety, although boundaries for safety will depend on whether the specific safety concerns (e.g., death) can be prespecified. Efficacy boundaries are often prespecified, but it is less common to prespecify safety boundaries due to the ad hoc nature of safety signals, especially in phase III trials.

For adaptive trials, especially for those that are "less well-understood," such as adaptive dose-finding decisions, seamless phase 2/3 designs, and unblinded adaptive sample size reestimation procedures, special expertise on the DMC could be required to make adaptive decisions (FDA draft guidance 2006, 2010). In such scenarios, often both efficacy and safety will be monitored. Adaptive designs also include the potential that certain decisions may inadvertently unblind study participants, and it is unclear whether or not a sponsor should be involved in the adaptive decision-making (Gallo 2006a,b).

Other issues include the potential conflict between an adaptive decision, typically based on efficacy data, and the accumulating safety data being reviewed by the DMC (Herson 2008, 2009). DMCs are further discussed in Section 8.3.2.1.

8.3 Adverse Event Monitoring

The National Institutes of Health require data and safety monitoring, generally, in the form of DMC or Data and Safety Monitoring Boards (DSMBs) for phase III clinical trials. For earlier trials (phase I and phase II), a DSMB may be appropriate if the studies have multiple clinical sites, are blinded (masked), or employ particularly high-risk interventions or vulnerable populations; otherwise, safety monitoring can be performed by a study investigator or a study safety team. A formal stopping rule for toxicity can serve as a useful reference for a DSMB or a safety monitoring team when reviewing the totality of toxicity data in oncology trials.

Phase I trials in oncology are conducted among cancer patients, typically with an assumption that the benefit of the cancer treatment will increase with the dose. The severity of toxicity is also expected to increase with the dose, so the challenge is to increase the dose without causing an unacceptable toxicity to patients. The goal of phase I trials is to identify the maximum tolerated dose (MTD). Phase II studies are conducted at the MTD estimated from phase I, and they evaluate whether a new drug has sufficient efficacy to warrant further development and refine the knowledge of its safety profile. In phase II trials, the toxicity rule can be developed to evaluate if the trial needs to be stopped early due to levels of toxicity higher than expected. Phase III trials examine the BR trade-off to determine if the trial needs to be stopped. The safety objectives of phase I trials are discussed in Chapter 1 of this book; we limit our discussion of safety monitoring to phase II and phase III clinical trials in this chapter. Since the occurrence of clinically relevant changes in other safety endpoints are often reported as AEs, the primary focus of this section is AE monitoring.

8.3.1 Toxicity Monitoring in Single-Arm Phase II Trials

The goal of a phase II oncology clinical study is to gain preliminary insights into the clinical activity of a novel treatment regimen. Most contemporary phase II oncology trials are single-arm or non-comparative multi-arm studies (Ivanova et al. 2016), with efficacy as a primary endpoint and toxicity as a secondary endpoint. Phase I oncology trials are designed to assess the toxicity of novel therapies. However, given the relatively small number of patients in phase I oncology trials, the recommended phase II dose can be imprecisely defined, leading to excessive toxicity in a phase II trial. Additionally, the patient characteristics in phase I can differ from the patients enrolled in a phase II trial (e.g., patients with solid cancer tumors vs patients with a specific type of cancer). Most phase II trials are designed to terminate a study early if the treatment is not promising for further development. It is equally important in a phase II oncology trial to not only have stopping rules for efficacy or a lack of therefore but also have stopping rules for toxicity.

Frequentist and Bayesian methods have been developed to evaluate both toxicity and efficacy as bivariate (efficacy, safety) variables. Most methods are two-stage and range from an equal weighting of efficacy response and toxicity to designs with variable trade-offs between these two outcomes. For example, the designs of Conaway and Petroni (1995), and Bryant and Day (1995) extend the two-stage Simon's designs by considering a new agent sufficiently promising if it exhibits both a response rate higher than the standard therapy and a toxicity rate that does not exceed the current standard of care. Conaway and Petroni (1996) proposed a trade-off design between response and toxicity rates that permits the level of toxicity to increase according to the observed response rate. Thall, Simon, and Estey (1995, 1996), Thall and Sung (1998), Thall and Cheng (1999), Chen and Smith (2009), and Thall (2008) proposed Bayesian methods for the simultaneous monitoring of both response and toxicity that allow for trade-offs between efficacy and toxicity rates.

Case Study 1 (Interim Stopping For Excessive Toxicity)

A phase II study examined a systemic anticancer therapy consisting of oxaliplatin, infusional 5-fluorouracil, and cetuximab concurrent with external beam irradiation prior to definitive esophagectomy in patients with operable esophageal adenocarcinoma (Gibson et al. 2010). A Simon two-stage design (Simon 1989) was used with a complete pathologic response as the primary endpoint. Toxicity was an important secondary endpoint and was monitored closely with monthly teleconferences, but there was no formal stopping rule for toxicity in the study protocol. By the time 22 patients were enrolled and treated, 6 treatment-related deaths (grade 5 toxicity) were observed. The study was stopped early for excessive toxicity. Standard multimodality therapy, namely, the regimen without cetuximab, is also associated with a known significant AE profile. However, the number of deaths of the experimental therapy was much higher than expected.

It is recommended to have a formal stopping rule to terminate the trial early for toxicity. One possibility is to have a single interim analysis; however, evaluating toxicity formally only once during the trial may not be sufficient. Does observing three treatment-related deaths in the first five patients warrant stopping the trial? A question like this might be raised by DSMB. Therefore, it might be beneficial to have a stopping rule that is continuous; that is, monitoring occurs throughout the study and stopping boundary is specified for each n, where n is the number of patients. For each n, the rule specifies the minimum number of toxicities that warrant stopping the study out of the total number of patients who have already been enrolled and have completed their follow-up for toxicity. For example, if investigators anticipate approximately 5% of deaths within the study, a potential formal stopping rule (Pocock 1977) would recommend trial suspension if at least two grade 5 events are observed in the first 2–4 patients, at least three events are observed in 5–12 patients, at least four events in 13–21 patients, at least five events in 22–31 patients, and if six or more events are observed in more than 31 patients.

A safety stopping rule can be based on frequentist or Bayesian approaches. Frequentists use fixed parameters to describe the unknown state of truth. Bayesian approaches take into account the accumulated information from prior experience (the *prior*), as well as the data collected (the *likelihood function*), to update and adapt the trial design (Berry 2012). We describe stopping rules based on frequentist and Bayesian approaches.

8.3.1.1 Frequentist Stopping Boundaries in Phase II

Consider a hypothetical example of an oncology phase II trial with a total sample size of 20. To define a stopping rule for excessive dose-limiting toxicities (DLTs) for this study, one needs to specify an acceptable probability for observing a DLT, θ_0. Usually, θ_0 is the target probability of a DLT in the corresponding phase I trial. Since most oncology phase I trials use the 3 + 3 design, the target DLT probability is often 0.20 or 0.25 (Reiner et al. 1999).

The two most frequently used boundaries are the O'Brien–Fleming (OBF) (O'Brien and Fleming 1979) and the Pocock (Pocock 1977) boundaries (columns 5 and 6, Table 8.1). The OBF boundary achieves higher power compared to the Pocock boundary for a given sample size and type-I error rate (α). That is, when used for the sequential monitoring of toxicity, the OBF boundary will yield a higher probability of stopping the trial for excessive toxicity when the toxicity is indeed excessive compared to the Pocock boundary. However, the Pocock boundary will stop the trial earlier than the OBF boundary, and, therefore, will yield less observed toxicities on average compared to the OBF boundary. For example, as shown in Table 8.1, if the Pocock boundary is used, the trial will stop if three DLTs are observed in the first three patients. In comparison, if the OBF boundary is used, the earliest stopping point requires that the first six patients all experience DLTs. Both boundaries shown in Table 8.1 have the probability of stopping the trial at $\alpha = 0.05$, the type-I error rate, if the toxicity probability is tolerable, that is, $\theta_0 = 0.2$.

The Pocock stopping rule can alternatively be described as repeated testing of the probability of toxicity after each patient completes toxicity follow-up, with the null hypothesis that the DLT probability is equal to $\theta_0 = 0.2$ and a type-I error rate α'. The point-wise α-level, α', is much

TABLE 8.1

Stopping Boundaries for a Trial with 20 Patients

	Bayesian Boundary			OBF	Pocock		
Number of Patients	Beta(0.6, 2.4) $\tau = 0.98$	Beta(4, 16) $\tau = 0.98$	Beta(0.6, 2.4) $\tau = 0.911$	Multistage	Multistage	Two-Stage	Three-Stage
1	–	–	–	–	–	–	–
2	–	–	–	–	–	–	–
3	3	–	–	–	3	–	–
4	4	–	4	–	4	–	–
5	4	–	5	–	4	–	–
6	5	6	5	6	4	–	–
7	5	7	5	6	5	–	5
8	5	7	5	6	5	–	–
9	6	7	6	6	5	–	–
10	6	7	6	6	6	6	–
11	6	8	6	6	6	–	–
12	7	8	6	7	6	–	–
13	7	8	7	7	7	–	–
14	7	9	7	7	7	–	7
15	7	9	7	7	7	–	–
16	8	9	7	7	8	–	–
17	8	9	8	7	8	–	–
18	8	10	8	8	8	–	–
19	9	10	8	8	9	–	–
20	9	10	8	8	9	8	8

Stopping boundaries for a trial with 20 patients with acceptable DLT probability of $\theta_0 = 0.2$. The trial is stopped after k patients if the number of observed DLTs is equal to or higher than the corresponding value of the boundary. OBF: O'Brien-Fleming Boundary. The probability of stopping the trial when the toxicity rate is acceptable is 0.05 for all boundaries.

smaller than the overall type-I error rate and can be computed for a given α. In the Pocock stopping boundary in Table 8.1, the point-wise $\alpha' = 0.0196$ corresponds to $\alpha = 0.05$. Ivanova et al. (2005) provide a table of values α' for various sample sizes (n) and tolerable DLT probability θ_0. Free software to generate the Pocock stopping boundary is available at http://cancer.unc.edu/biostatistics/program/ivanova/. For given n, θ_0, and α, the software computes the stopping boundary and important quantities that describe the boundary's performance. For several values of the true DLT probability θ_0, the program computes the probability of stopping a trial and declaring that the therapy is too toxic, the average number of DLTs, and the average number of patients in the trial (Table 8.2). For example, when the probability of DLT is 0.4, about half of the trials are stopped (probability of stopping is 0.55). The software also provides an example write-up that can be used in clinical trial protocols.

TABLE 8.2

Operating Characteristics for a Trial with 20 Patients

True DLT Probability	Early Stopping Probability	Expected Number of DLTs	Expected Number of Enrolled Patients
0.2	0.05	3.9	19.5
0.4	0.55	5.8	14.6
0.5	0.83	5.4	10.8
0.6	0.97	4.7	7.8
0.8	1.00	3.6	4.5

Operating characteristics of the Pocock boundary with 20 patients, acceptable DLT probability of $\theta_0 = 0.2$, and the type-I error rate of 0.05.

8.3.1.2 Bayesian Stopping Boundaries in Phase II

To compute a frequentist boundary, a tolerable level of toxicity ($\theta_0 = 0.2$), a type-I error rate ($\alpha = 0.05$), the shape of the boundary, for example, Pocock or OBF, and the total sample size (n) of the study are required. To compute a Bayesian stopping boundary, we need to specify a tolerable level of DLT ($\theta_0 = 0.2$), the prior distribution for the DLT probability, and the tolerance cutoff, τ. The Beta distribution is used as a prior for DLT probability, requiring the specification of the distribution parameters a and b. For example, the prior $Beta(a = 2, b = 8)$ can be viewed as reflecting the prior information from 10 patients (2 experienced DLTs whereas 8 did not) who were, for example, enrolled in a prior phase I trial. As data are being collected from the ongoing phase II trial, the posterior distribution is computed. For example, if 5 and 25 patients have completed the ongoing phase II trial with and without a DLT, respectively, the posterior distribution of the probability of a DLT is $Beta(2{+}5, 8{+}25)$, with a corresponding mean DLT probability of 0.21. According to the prior, the probability that the DLT rate was larger than 0.2 was 43%. After obtaining the data, this probability is 31%. On the other hand, if 10 DLTs are observed among these 30 patients, the posterior distribution of the probability of DLT is $Beta(2 + 10, 8 + 20)$. In this case, the DLT probability is estimated as 0.43, and the probability that the DLT rate is larger than 0.2 is now 93%.

Geller et al. (2005) proposed a Bayesian stopping rule for continuous monitoring of toxicity. The trial is stopped if the posterior probability of the DLT rate exceeding θ_0 is equal to or higher than a prespecified value τ, usually 0.90, 0.95, or 0.98. The rule is continuous as it checks whether or not the total number of observed DLTs is too high after DLT information becomes available on every new patient. Columns 2 and 3 of Table 8.1 provide two Bayesian stopping boundaries for a trial of a total of $n = 20$ patients and $\tau = 0.98$ for $\theta_0 = 0.2$. A stopping boundary is described by a set of integers b_k, $k = 1, \ldots, n$, such that the trial is stopped if there are b_k or more DLTs observed out of first k patients with complete toxicity follow-up. The prior distribution, the value of tolerable DLT probability θ_0, and the value of τ

uniquely define the set of integers b_k that can be computed prior to the start of the trial. To use the Bayesian boundary, there is no need to compute the probability that the DLT rate is larger than $\theta_0 = 0.2$ given the current data. Instead, one can simply check if the number of observed DLTs in the first k patients is equal to or exceeds b_k. The boundary in column 2 uses the prior *Beta*(0.6, 2.4), reflecting information from the total of 0.6 + 2.4 = 3 patients. The prior experience might reflect information from a 3-patient dose cohort or from a 6-patient dose cohort of a phase I trial. In the latter case, the prior experience was down-weighted from 6 to 3 patients, that is, *Beta*(0.6, 2.4) was used instead of *Beta*(1.2, 4.8). The overall probability of stopping the trial for the boundary in column 2 of Table 8.1 when the DLT rate is equal to the acceptable rate of 0.2 is 0.038. The boundary in column 3 of Table 8.1 uses the prior *Beta*(4, 16), which reflects information from 20 patients with an observed DLT probability of 4/20 = 0.20. Because there is strong prior information that the DLT probability is close to 0.20, stronger evidence is needed in the phase II trial that the DLT probability is high in order to stop the trial compared to the first boundary. This is also reflected in the very small overall probability (0.004) of stopping the trial when the DLT probability is equal to the acceptable DLT rate. The overall probability of stopping when the probability of toxicity is acceptable is a useful metric as it is the same as the frequentist type-I error rate. Column 4 of Table 8.1 shows a boundary with the prior *Beta*(4, 16) and $\tau = 0.911$ where the overall probability of stopping is 0.05 when the true toxicity probability is 0.2.

In general, and as seen from Table 8.1, the Bayesian boundary with the *Beta*(0.6, 2.4) prior and $\tau = 0.98$ is almost indistinguishable from the Pocock boundary. Less informative priors, that is, priors where $a + b$ from a *Beta* distribution is low, for example, 0.6 + 2.4 = 3, yield a Bayesian boundary similar to the Pocock boundary as long as the two boundaries yield a similar overall probability of stopping. In the case of informative priors, where $a + b$ is high, more DLTs are required to occur within the ongoing phase II trial to recommend trial interruption. More DLTs need to be observed to stop the phase II trial, because we need to override the prior information that the toxicity rate is tolerable. In the example shown in Table 8.1, under the Bayesian rule with an informative prior regarding the probability of stopping of 0.05 ($\tau = 0.911$), we stop later than under the Pocock boundary but earlier than the OBF boundary.

8.3.1.3 Two-Stage, Three-Stage, or Multistage Designs for Stopping for Toxicity in Phase II

Consider a two-stage Pocock boundary with a probability of stopping of at most 0.05 when toxicity probability is 0.2. According to the two-stage boundary, the trial is stopped if six or more DLTs are observed in the first 10 patients and if eight or more DLTs are observed in 20 patients, or equivalently, point-wise $\alpha' = 0.0325$ is used (Table 8.2). This boundary is a two-stage counterpart of the Pocock continuous boundary (column 7 in Table 8.1). Due to the discreteness of the binomial distribution, the decision rules for a two-stage boundary in this example are very similar to the corresponding rules in the 20-stage boundary: $\geq 6/10$ and $\geq 8/20$ for the two-stage, and $\geq 6/10$ and $\geq 9/20$ for the 20-stage boundary. The multistage boundary is more flexible as it allows stopping at many points of the trial. The expected number of DLTs before the trial is stopped if the two-stage boundary is used for true DLT probabilities of 0.4, 0.5, 0.6, and 0.8 are 7.3, 8.1, 8.3, and 8.3 compared to 5.8, 5.4, 4.7, and 3.6 for the continuous boundary (Table 8.2). That is, three more DLTs are observed on average if the two-stage boundary is used. The expected number of enrolled patients for the two-stage boundary is 18.3, 16.2, 13.7, and 10.3 compared to 14.6, 10.8, 7.8, and 4.5 for the continuous boundary (Table 8.2). For a three-stage boundary, the decision rules are $\geq 5/7, \geq 7/14$, and $\geq 8/20$ (column 8, Table 8.1). The rules coincide with the continuous boundary decision rules except at the last look. A multistage boundary allows exhausting the type-I error rate more effectively and efficiently. Examples of two-stage designs where a trial can be stopped after stage 1 because of high toxicity can be found in (Elter et al. 2005; Krug et al. 2005; Penson et al. 2010). A multistage design with interim analysis for toxicity after every 10 patients (or after every 20 patients) is discussed in (Brada et al. 2005; Ross et al. 2010).

Summary of recommendations for stopping for excessive toxicity in a phase II trial

- Keep the probability of stopping the trial when the DLT probability is equal to the acceptable DLT rate at 0.05 or lower regardless of whether the frequentist or the Bayesian boundary is used.
- Between the two frequentist stopping boundaries most commonly used in clinical trials, the Pocock boundary and the OBF boundary, we recommend the Pocock boundary because it allows stopping for toxicity as early as possible.
- If a Bayesian boundary is considered, a boundary with the prior centered around the acceptable DLT rate and a small effective sample size $(a + b)$ in the prior is similar to the Pocock boundary. If effective sample size $(a + b)$ in the prior is large, the boundary is similar to the OBF boundary.
- Use a multistage boundary rather than the two- or three-stage boundary. Due to discreetness of the binomial distribution, almost no power is lost when additional looks are added to the two- or three-stage boundary to make a multistage boundary.
- If it is likely that a large number of patients could be enrolled within a short period of time, it is recommended to employ an enrolment rule (Song and Ivanova 2015) to determine when to enroll patients or when to delay enrolment.

8.3.2 Toxicity Monitoring in Randomized Phase II and Phase III Clinical Trials

In the assessment of the BR balance in oncology, the weight given to more common AEs affecting tolerability versus infrequent severe or life-threatening AEs differs depending on the disease stage and setting (EMA 2016). In the palliative setting, good tolerability may be given priority; also, in a curative setting, tolerability may be given less emphasis as long as it does not compromise the completion of therapy. In the palliative setting, infrequent severe or even fatal AEs may be considered to be an acceptable risk, but in the adjuvant setting, where therapy is given based on an assumption that many patients would be cured by the prior surgery alone and even more with the standard adjuvant therapy, the acceptance of life-threatening AEs is generally lower. The BR assessment in the neoadjuvant setting is more complex, as it depends largely on the operability of the tumor. Higher risks may be acceptable for treatments in patients with primarily inoperable tumors, such as locally advanced or metastatic cancer.

The primary endpoints in randomized phase II and phase III clinical trials in oncology are usually overall survival (OS), progression-free survival, or disease-free survival (DFS). All of these endpoints include death as an outcome, but stopping rules for a primary endpoint does not cover situations when unexpected or highly significant events other than death emerge in safety. Additionally, safety reviews are usually conducted more often than interim analyses for efficacy to stop a trial as soon as possible if unexpected severe toxicity is observed, though the continuous safety monitoring described in Section 8.3.1 might not be realistic in large multisite randomized phase II and phase III oncology trials. For most randomized studies, safety monitoring is done by an independent DSMB at preplanned safety analyses.

The Pocock, OBF, or Bayesian boundaries can be used to monitor toxicity in randomized phase II and phase III clinical trials (Lewis and Berry 1994; Jennison and Turnbull 2000; Berry et al. 2011). Generally, the BR trade-off is evaluated to decide if the trial needs to be stopped due to toxicity and the decision is primarily based on qualitative approaches and the expert judgment (DSMB). For readers interested in qualitative and quantitative BR assessment methods, we recommend Jiang and He (2016).

8.3.2.1 Independent Committees to Review Safety Data

Data and safety monitoring in clinical trials can be defined as a planned, ongoing process of reviewing the data collected in a clinical trial with the primary purpose of protecting the safety of trial participants, the credibility of the trial, and the validity of trial results (Ellenberg et al. 2002; Dixon et al. 2006). As mentioned in Section 8.2.2, independent DSMB is usually responsible for data and safety monitoring in randomized phase II and phase III studies. Sometimes safety reviews occur with the same frequency as efficacy reviews, but more frequent safety meetings are typical practice. How often should the DSMB review the data? The answer depends on how fast the information becomes available. Most oncology DSMBs meet and review safety data every 6 months (Green et al. 2003), though annual monitoring is recommended for adjuvant therapy or slower accruing trials. Safety monitoring can be blinded or unblinded. For interim safety review of randomized trials, DSMB members usually receive reports with partially blinded or masked treatment groups. In this case, patient data is summarized by the actual treatment group, with the groups labeled as A and B, where the meaning of A and B is not disclosed to the DSMB members unless specifically requested. Blinded monitoring of individual safety data is usually performed by the study team or the study coordinator. The DSMB may request unblinded summaries of efficacy in addition to safety when the study under review is considered for early termination due to a safety concern.

In guidance for clinical trial sponsors on Establishment and Operation of Clinical Trial Data Monitoring Committees (2006), the United States Food and Drug Administration (US FDA) defined a clinical trial DMC as "a group of individuals with pertinent expertise that reviews on a regular basis accumulating data from one or more ongoing clinical trials." They note that a DMC is also known as a DSMB or a Data and Safety Monitoring Committee (DSMC). Because different expertise and experience may be necessary to make appropriate recommendations, questions sometimes arise as to whether some trials, for example, adaptive trials, should have a single DMC or two committees—DMC and DSMB—one that can address efficacy adaptations and the other one that can meet more often to review the safety data more thoroughly (Antonijevic et al. 2013). We recommend a single committee, with members possessing the relevant expertise and experience necessary for the interim review and decision-making to avoid confusion or conflicts in recommendations between multiple groups. While two committees responsible for the oversight of one clinical trial makes the review process more complicated, it could be acceptable if the responsibilities and the communication process are clearly outlined upfront. Very often, industry-sponsored clinical programs utilize the same independent DMC for all trials in a development program, sometimes going as far as possible for multiple programs for a compound under investigation. Although DMC decisions are advisory, they should be taken seriously by company executives responsible for the study validity and integrity.

In the draft guidance for industry on Safety Assessment for IND Safety Reporting (2015), the US FDA recommends that sponsors use a safety assessment committee. This safety assessment committee should oversee "the evolving safety profile of the investigational drug by evaluating, at appropriate intervals, the cumulative serious adverse events (SAEs) from all of the trials in the development program, as well as other available important safety information (e.g., findings from epidemiological studies and from animal or in vitro testing) and performing unblinded comparisons of event rates in investigational and control groups, as needed, so the sponsor may meet its obligations under § 312.32(b) and (c)." The safety assessment committee is distinct from a DMC with different roles and operational practices. In most cases, an existing DMC will not be able to function as a safety assessment committee because the DMC may meet too infrequently and is often focused on a single trial, rather than the entire safety database. Further, DMCs recommend to the sponsor when to modify or stop a study because the investigational drug is ineffective or exhibits an important safety concern. In contrast, the role of the safety assessment committee is to review accumulating safety data to determine when to recommend that the sponsor submit an IND safety report to the FDA and investigators participating in the clinical program. Despite their distinct roles, the safety assessment committee can participate with a DMC for decisions as to whether the conduct of a specific study should be revised based on the currently available safety information.

8.3.2.2 Examples of Early Stopping in Oncology Trials

There are many examples of clinical studies stopped early in oncology. Reasons for stopping trials early include stopping for positive results including good efficacy and acceptable toxicity, or negative results including futility (inability to distinguish from a control), unacceptable toxicity, or slow patient enrolment. We summarize some important case studies and discuss the impact of early trial termination.

Case Study 2 (Emergency stopping based on unexpected toxic death)

The Southwest oncology group (SWOG) study 9028 (Samon et al. 1998, Green et al. 2003) was designed to test the hypothesis that the standard therapy plus agents to block the transport of drugs from cells would be more effective than the standard therapy alone in the treatment of multiple myeloma. Patients were randomized to receive either vincristine, doxorubicin, and dexamethasone (VAD) or VAD plus VQ (verapamil and quinine) to overcome multidrug resistance. The difficulty in the evaluation of multiple myeloma patients is the determination of the cause of death. Patients who die due to the disease often die of multiple organ failure, which makes it difficult to distinguish death due to disease from death due to organ toxicities. Shortly after SWOG 9028 was open to accrual, several deaths of patients treated with VAD plus VQ were reported. The study coordinator reviewed the information and judged that these deaths were due to renal failure in patients with poor renal function at diagnosis and were possibly related to verapamil. An amendment to the protocol was prepared to reduce the dose of verapamil in patients with poor renal function and the DMC was notified. By the time of the scheduled DMC meeting, the evidence of toxic death from verapamil was stronger and even though the survival differences were not statistically significant, the VAD plus VQ treatment arm was closed to further accrual. Later, all patients treated with VAD plus VQ were taken off verapamil.

Even though the DSMB was established to review safety data at prespecified times, it was obvious that the blinded review by a study coordinator was important to take an appropriate course of action since the observed safety result could not wait until the semiannual DSMB meeting. Had the study coordinator waited until the formal DSMB meeting, more patients would have died due to toxicity. It is important for the study team or the study coordinator to perform a blinded review of safety data regularly. Reducing the doses of experimental or even standard treatments in oncology trials is a standard approach to address observed safety concerns. Very often, a study protocol outlines AEs and toxicity grades that, if observed, would lead to a dose reduction. It allows a patient to continue the study with an assumption of reduced toxicity. However, it is very rare that statistical analyses of the data account for these dose reductions.

Case Study 3 (Stopping early for negative results)

This was a trial of high-dose cisplatin with or without mitomycin C versus a control arm of standard-dose cisplatin in patients with advanced non–small cell lung cancer (Gandara et al. 1993, Green et al. 2003). The trial was supposed to enroll about 200 patients per treatment arm to achieve a power of 82.5% to detect a hazard ratio of 1.25. Interim analyses were planned at about 33% and 66% of the expected information at one-sided 0.005 levels. At the first interim analysis (at about 50% of the planned accrual), the alternative hypothesis for the comparison of high-dose to standard-dose cisplatin was rejected with a p-value of 0.003. Even though neither the null nor the alternative hypothesis of the high-dose cisplatin plus mitomycin C could have been rejected, the rationale for the use of high-dose cisplatin was called into question. Additionally, two high-dose cisplatin arms had significantly more toxicity than the standard-dose arm. The DMC decided that the trial should be closed at this point. The results were still negative at the time of publication.

This is an example of the DMC review of data using the BR approach—taking into account the benefit (or lack of benefit in this case) and the accompanying risk to decide whether to stop the study or not. One of the criticisms in this example was that the trial was terminated early for unconvincing results. Stopping early for unconvincing negative results can have serious consequences, especially for other ongoing trials involving the same treatment. There are more examples of trials that were negative but inconclusive and stopped early (Green et al. 2003). In the case when a similar trial (SWOG 9623) was underway and inconclusive results from another trial were presented, the patient recruitment to the ongoing trial diminished and the trial was eventually closed due to poor accrual. The question as to whether chemotherapy was valuable for this patient population was not answered.

Case Study 4 (Stopping early for positive results)

This was a randomized phase III trial in early breast cancer (George and Green 2006) coordinated by the Cancer and Leukemia Group B, with participation by SWOG, the Eastern Cooperative Oncology Group, and the North Central Cancer Treatment Group. The trial was designed as a factorial design to evaluate three different doses of doxorubicin with and without paclitaxel added to standard chemotherapy (3 × 2 factorial design). It was already established that adjuvant chemotherapy was important in extending survival in patients with early breast cancer. In particular, the use of an alkylating agent together with doxorubicin was known to be beneficial. However, there was uncertainty regarding optimal drug dosing (doxorubicin had significant cardiac toxicity at higher cumulative doses), the patient population who might benefit the most from the therapy, and the role of paclitaxel in the adjuvant setting. To address these questions, a randomized clinical trial CALGP 9344 was designed and activated in 1994. DFS and OS were the primary endpoints. At least two administrative analyses took place together with the toxicity reports review (safety analyses) prior to the first formal efficacy analysis. Originally, there were no formal rules for interim analyses for efficacy, though they were later added per request from the DMC. The protocol was modified to include three interim efficacy analyses at 450, 900, and 1,350 events and a final analysis at 1,800 events (at 25%, 50%, 75%, and at 100% of expected events). The first formal efficacy analysis took place at 453 events (approximately at 25% of planned events). At this time, the trial was closed to accrual for about a year and all patients had been off all protocol treatment for at least six months. As in the previous administrative analyses, the DFS outcome appeared to favor the paclitaxel treatment group, although the nominal significance level still failed to reach the prespecified monitoring OBF boundary. At this point, the DMC decided to release the results to the sponsoring community, and the results were shared at a special ASCO session shortly thereafter. Four years later and five years after the study recruitment was closed, the second analysis at 1,054 events (approximately at 58% of expected events) was performed. This analysis supported the previous decision, with the OBF boundary crossed. It was the last formal analysis.

This is an example of the DSMB decision on efficacy most likely driven by the observed positive trend in unblinded efficacy data at the preplanned safety analyses (the so-called administrative looks, when unblinded results are presented but there is no intent to make a decision with regard to efficacy). Safety appeared to have not been an issue at the time when the DSMB made a decision to stop the study for positive results. The trial was closed to accrual for about a year, and all ongoing patients had been off all protocol treatment for at least six months. More detailed discussions on issues such as the effect on patients enrolled in the study, the effect on the medical and research community, stopping rules versus stopping guidelines, crossovers, statistical predictions, early versus late outcomes, and the role of the DSMB in this study can be found in George and Green 2006. Here, we would like to discuss the role of repetitive exposure of DSMB members to administrative ("non-actionable") interim analyses in detail. In George et al. (2004), the authors discuss whether there is a danger for DMC members in slipping from objective stewards of the study data to advocate for a specific interpretation of the findings. A survey was administered to 21 DMC members to investigate how they evaluated accumulating evidence. The results indicated that some DMC members may overinterpret developing results in the data. Administrative looks at efficacy data should not be performed at the preplanned safety analyses. One opinion is that both safety and efficacy analyses should be performed at the same time with a flexible α-spending approach for efficacy. For example, the timing of interim analyses is not an issue if a spending function approach is used. If there is no intention to stop a study very early for efficacy because of the lack of sufficient information on safety or a long-term efficacy, but the unblinded analysis is performed for both safety and efficacy, the α allocated to control the type-I error to test efficacy at interim analyses should be very small. This opinion is driven perhaps by an idea of performing a more structured BR assessment at each interim look or to just avoid questions on the possibility of a non-penalized unblinded look at efficacy. In this case, the issue discussed by George et al. (2004) might still exist, especially, when the decisions are based on a synthesis of statistical methodology and clinical judgment. Another approach would drop administrative looks at efficacy entirely at interim safety analyses. If there is a serious safety issue that calls for data on endpoints to decide whether a study needs to be stopped early, then a flexible α-spending approach for efficacy can be performed.

All three trials described as case studies were closed prior to the planned completion. The reasons for closing these studies were different: toxic death (safety), negative results (efficacy and safety), and positive results (good efficacy) when safety was not an issue. In the next section, we briefly discuss the consequences of aggressive stopping rules, driven primarily by efficacy.

8.3.2.3 Consequences of Aggressive Stopping Rules

The European Medicine Agency (EMA) and the US FDA allow sponsors to file for accelerated and conditional approvals for serious conditions (FDA guidance 2014; EMA guideline 2016). This led to a simplified and shortened process of development of a new drug, particularly in oncology. Interim analyses pose an ethical dilemma of safeguarding the interests of patients enrolled in clinical trials, while simultaneously protecting society from premature claims of treatment benefits. Trials that are stopped early because of safety or futility tend to result in prompt discontinuation of useless or potentially harmful interventions. In contrast, trials that are stopped early for benefit may result in the fast approval and dissemination of promising new treatments. Given the serious and life-threatening nature of cancer and patients' expectations, quicker clinical drug development is required. However, this may lead to a poorly defined BR of new therapies. Of particular concern has been the early stopping of trials when early efficacy endpoints (such as DFS or time to recurrence) are positive or the early stopping of trials with delayed toxicity. This has precluded any opportunity of clearly establishing overall benefit.

Trotta et al. (2008) discussed whether stopping a trial early in oncology is performed for the patients or for the industry. The authors reviewed 93 oncology clinical trials that had been stopped at interim analyses and noticed a consistent increase in prematurely stopped trials. They argued that there is a market-driven intent to sparing patients and saving time and trial costs. Montori et al. (2005) performed a systematic review of randomized trials that stopped early for benefit. The authors urged clinicians to interpret randomized clinical trials that stopped early for benefit with caution as the large treatment effect observed might be due to chance. Pocock (2005) comments on the Montori et al. paper and provides some insights on when (and when not) to stop a clinical trial for benefit. He suggests that decisions of early stopping should be based on wise judgments interpreting the totality of available evidence, both in the current trial (considering primary and other efficacy outcomes and safety issues) and from other sources of external evidence (especially from related trials). Pocock suggests that a statistical stopping boundary is only one useful objective component in an inevitably more challenging decision-making process. Paradoxically, the early stopping of trials with apparently successful outcomes can delay full approval of the treatment. Further, not observing a clear benefit of a new treatment might result in rejection or just partial reimbursement of the treatment by payers that could also lead to a new drug being not at all or hardly adapted by the medical community.

8.4 Reporting Safety

8.4.1 Data Collection and Summary

Gaining a clear picture for the safety of any drug can be challenging, but when the necessary understanding of patient safety is at its greatest, as it is in oncology, sufficient insight into the tolerability of a treatment is often more difficult to attain. Given the volume and complexity of the data available for safety outcomes, efficient and informative reporting is crucial to communicate patient well-being. In this section, we provide guidance on reporting safety in clinical trials of oncology, in trials with two or more arms, with a primary focus on AEs. Analyses of death and disease progression, while important indicators of patient safety, are typically the primary endpoints in oncology trials, and are covered in sufficient detail elsewhere in this book. Limited analyses for other safety endpoints, such as laboratory abnormalities, are also presented here. The interpretation of safety assessments from single-arm trials is challenging since many of the observed events are naturally occurring due to the underlying disease. In these situations, comparisons of the safety outcomes to historical information are required to understand any safety signals attributable to the drug.

Our rationale for the focus on AEs is due to the fact that occurrences of clinically relevant changes in other safety endpoints are often reported as AEs. For example, significant changes in the laboratory test alanine aminotransferase (ALT), an important indicator of liver health, can be represented by the AEs "ALT abnormal," "ALT increased," or "ALT decreased" when using the MedDRA dictionary (Brown et al. 1999). Despite our limited discussion of other safety endpoints, many of the recommendations made still apply. We illustrate the various methodologies using data from hematologic and solid tumor clinical trials of imatinib (Tables 8.3 and 8.4; MetaGIST 2010; Kantarjian et al. 2010; Novartis Pharmaceutical Corporation 2015).

Guideline E2A from the International Conference on Harmonization (ICH) defines an AE as "any untoward medical occurrence in a patient or clinical investigation subject administered a pharmaceutical product and which does not necessarily have to have a causal relationship with this treatment" (ICH 1994). Additionally, SAEs are AEs that "result in death, are life-threatening, require inpatient hospitalization or prolongation of hospitalization, result in disability or permanent damage, or are congenital anomalies or birth defects" (ICH 1994). Guidelines from the EMA define the additional term adverse drug reaction (ADR) for those events that are viewed by the investigator to have a causal relationship with treatment (EMA 2016). Adverse events that occur since the previous study visit are reported to the clinician by the patient or caregiver. Details on the toxicity grade (defined using the National Cancer Institute's Common Terminology Criteria of Adverse Events, NCI-CTCAE), seriousness, outcome, and duration of the event, along with the action taken with the study drug in response to the event, and the investigator's opinion on the relationship to study medication are recorded. The verbatim text is coded using a medical dictionary such as MedDRA, to maintain consistency in the reporting of AEs within and across studies and development programs (Brown et al. 1999). MedDRA further groups related events within a five-level hierarchy. AEs are traditionally summarized by preferred terms and are grouped by system organ class (SOC) in order of decreasing frequency of occurrence. For example, Table 8.3 summarizes (without SOC) drug-related AEs that occurred in at least 10% of treated patients from a clinical trial comparing dasatinib to imatinib for patients in newly diagnosed chronic-phase chronic myeloid leukemia (Kantarjian et al. 2010). Similar displays are often presented for the subset of events determined to be ADRs, with additional summaries of AEs and ADRs limited to those events with NCI-CTCAE grades 3 and above. Binary outcomes, such as whether a patient experienced a particular AE or not, are often reported using a risk difference ($\hat{p}_{tj} - \hat{p}_{cj}$), risk ratio ($\hat{p}_{tj}/\hat{p}_{cj}$), or odds ratio $\left(\hat{p}_{tj}\left(1-\hat{p}_{cj}\right)/\left(1-\hat{p}_{tj}\right)\hat{p}_{cj}\right)$, where $\hat{p}_{ij}$ is the probability of experiencing event j of J possible AEs for treatment i (Chuang-Stein et al. 2014; Zhou et al. 2015). Risk differences are presented throughout this section (e.g., Table 8.3, Figures 8.2–8.4). Pros and cons for the various measures are discussed in Zhou et al. (2015).

Given the large number of potential comparisons of treatment arms for AEs, Crowe and coauthors suggested a three-tier approach for the analysis of AEs (Crowe et al. 2009). Preplanned hypothesis for Tier I events, those AEs expected to occur or those of considerable clinical relevance for the disease (the AESIs defined in Section 8.2.1), would typically not receive adjustments for multiple comparisons unless there were numerous Tier I events. Further, they recommended that the detection of important differences among commonly occurring (in four or more patients in a single treatment arm), though unexpected AEs should consider multiple comparisons (Tier II). Tier III events (those not in Tiers I or II) should be summarized in a listing. Appropriate multiplicity adjustment for Tier I (if necessary) and Tier II events should achieve a reasonable balance between committing type-I errors without overly sacrificing the power to detect potential safety signals. The false discovery rate (FDR) method provides a more balanced approach between type-I error and power, since it does not control the familywise error rate (Benjamini and Hochberg 1995). Among the rejected null hypotheses from a family of multiple tests, the proportion of erroneous rejections, typically controlled at a prespecified α of 0.05, is defined as the FDR. In general, with J treatment comparisons of ordered (smallest to largest) p-values $p_{(j)}$, the FDR p-value for the jth hypothesis is

$$p_{(j)}^{*} = \begin{cases} p_{(J)} & \text{for } j = J \\ \min\left(p_{(j)}^{*}, \dfrac{j}{(j-1)} p_{(j-1)}\right) & \text{for } j = 1, 2, \ldots (J-1) \end{cases}.$$

Corresponding simultaneous 95% FDR confidence intervals can be defined by finding the largest j where $p_{(j)} \le j\alpha/J$ and using $\alpha^{*} = j\alpha/J$ for all J confidence intervals (Benjamini and Yekutieli 2005). Table 8.3 presents unadjusted and FDR-adjusted p-values for Fisher's exact test and unadjusted and FDR-adjusted 95% confidence intervals for the dasatinib minus imatinib risk difference using the normal approximation to the binomial. An alternate FDR methodology that considers the relationship among AEs, the double FDR, could also be considered for analysis (Mehrotra and Adewale 2012).

All of the information needed to understand the safety of the treatments is available in Table 8.3, but the message is not communicated very well. Alternatively, a volcano plot (Figure 8.1) can be used to summarize the

TABLE 8.3

Drug-Related AEs that Occurred in at Least 10% of Treated Patients

Preferred Term	Dasatinib ($N = 258$)	Imatinib ($N = 258$)	Unadjusted 95% Confidence Interval and p-value	FDR Confidence Interval and p-value
Anemia	232 (90)	217 (84)	6 (0.2, 11.8) 0.0661	6 (–1.5, 13.5) 0.1074
Thrombocytopenia	181 (70)	160 (62)	8 (–0.1, 16.1) 0.0628	8 (–2.5, 18.5) 0.1074
Neutropenia	168 (65)	150 (58)	7 (–1.4, 15.4) 0.1237	7 (–3.8, 17.8) 0.1787
Fluid retention	49 (19)	108 (42)	–23 (–30.7, –15.3) <0.0001	–23 (–32.9, –13.1) <0.0001
Diarrhea	44 (17)	44 (17)	0 (–6.5, 6.5) 1.00	0 (–8.4, 8.4) 1.00
Nausea	21 (8)	52 (20)	–12 (–17.9, –6.1) 0.0001	–12 (–19.6, –4.4) 0.0005
Rash	28 (11)	44 (17)	–6 (–12.0, 0.0) 0.0561	–6 (–13.7, 1.7) 0.1074
Musculoskeletal pain	28 (11)	36 (14)	–3 (–8.7, 2.7) 0.3499	–3 (–10.4, 4.4) 0.4549
Headache	31 (12)	26 (10)	2 (–3.4, 7.4) 0.5746	2 (–5.0, 9.0) 0.6225
Muscle inflammation	10 (4)	44 (17)	–13 (–18.2, –7.8) <0.0001	–13 (–19.7, –6.3) <0.0001
Fatigue	21 (8)	26 (10)	–2 (–6.9, 2.9) 0.5409	–2 (–8.4, 4.4) 0.6225
Myalgia	15 (6)	31 (12)	–6 (–10.9, –1.1) 0.0196	–6 (–12.3, 0.3) 0.0638
Vomiting	13 (5)	26 (10)	–5 (–9.5, –0.5) 0.0445	–5 (–10.8, 0.8) 0.1074

Values are N(%). N was derived from % and arm totals. Data for treatment sample sizes and percentages from Table 4 of Kantarjian et al. (2010). Table is sorted by overall incidence of each event. Data on SOCs were not available. Confidence intervals are based on the risk difference of dasatinib minus imatinib using a normal approximation. For the FDR intervals, $\alpha^* = 3/13 \times 0.05 = 0.0115$.

incidence of AEs (Jin et al. 2001; Zink et al. 2013). The x-axis represents the dasatinib minus imatinib risk difference, while the y-axis represents the –log10 transformation of the unadjusted p-value from Fisher's exact test. The smaller the p-value, the larger the value on the y-axis; y can be thought of as the number of decimal places or the number of zeros in the p-value derived from the comparison of risk between the treatments. Bubble area is proportional to the total number of AEs that occur for both treatments combined. References lines are drawn to show significant events with no adjustment (–log10(0.05) = 1.3) or FDR adjustment (–log10(0.0115) = 1.9393, where $\alpha^* = 3/13 \times 0.05 = 0.0115$); events are significant if the center of the bubble

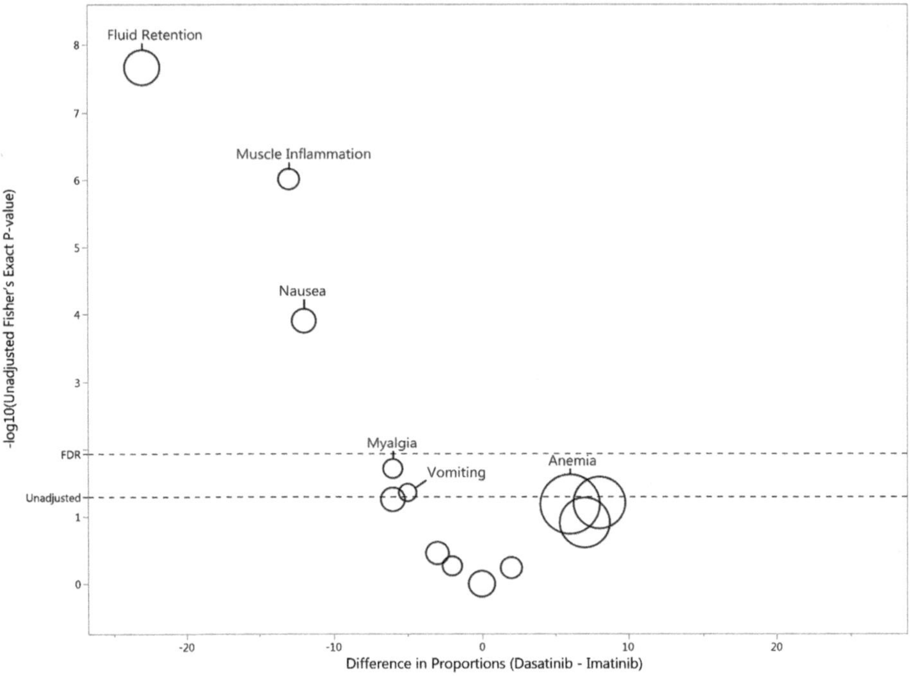

FIGURE 8.1
Volcano plot of drug-related AEs that occurred in at least 10% of the treated patients. Unadjusted reference line drawn at –log10(0.05) = 1.3. FDR reference line drawn at –log10(0.0115) = 1.9393, where $\alpha^* = 3/13 \times 0.05 = 0.0115$. Alternatively, the FDR reference line could be drawn at –log10(maximum unadjusted p-value $\leq\alpha^*$) as in Zink et al. (2013). Bubble area is proportional to the total number of AEs that occur for both treatments combined.

is above a particular reference line. Figure 8.1 communicates very clearly that anemia and vomiting are the most and least common events of Table 8.3; imatinib shows significantly greater unadjusted risk for fluid retention, muscle inflammation, nausea, myalgia, and vomiting; imatinib shows significantly greater FDR-adjusted risk for fluid retention, muscle inflammation, and nausea; and that the events with greater risk (though not statistically so) on dasatinib are very common. With the availability of color, bubbles could be colored according to Tier, SOC, or average toxicity grade to communicate additional information. See Zink et al. (2013) for suggestions on using volcano plots for other measures, statistical tests, and the reporting of risk over time. For trials in oncology, volcano plots utilizing cycle as a timescale help communicate ADRs that resolve over time as a tolerance to study medication develops. On the other hand, events that occur due to the cumulative toxicity of study treatments will become readily apparent as the trial progresses. Further, EMA guidance suggests presentations of cumulative AE rates at 3, 6, and 12 months, with the addition of other time points depending on the underlying nature of the disease and the duration of the trial (EMA 2016).

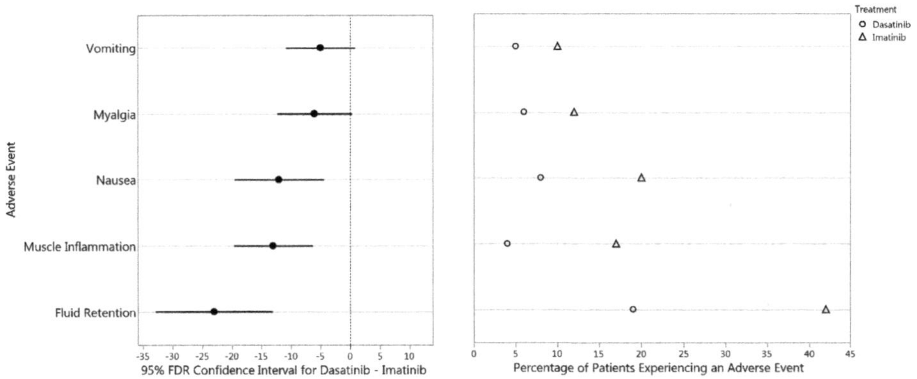

FIGURE 8.2
FDR intervals and event incidence for identified safety signals. The presentation is suggested as in Amit et al. (2008). The left panel displays a forest plot (Lewis and Clarke 2001) of FDR intervals for dasatinib minus imatinib for signals identified in Figure 8.1. The reference line is drawn at 0 to indicate no difference between dasatinib and imatinib. Right panel presents a dot plot to communicate the incidence of each AE for each treatment arm.

To communicate additional details for important events identified from the volcano plot, Figure 8.2 summarizes FDR intervals and incidence rates using a forest plot and a dot plot (Lewis and Clarke 2001; Amit et al. 2008).

8.4.2 Subgroups

Subgroups are frequently considered for the analysis of safety and efficacy endpoints, with 70% of clinical trials reporting at least some results within subgroups (Pocock et al. 2002). Subgroup analyses are beneficial in that they provide clinicians with information on the potential for differential treatment response within important demographic, genetic, disease, environmental, behavioral, or regional characteristics (Quan et al. 2010; Chuang-Stein et al. 2014). From a regulatory perspective, such analyses are important to show that the estimated overall effect is broadly applicable to patients and to assess risk-benefit across the proposed indication, particularly when the study population is heterogeneous (CHMP 2014). Further, examining results within subgroups allows the study team to assess the consistency and robustness of results obtained for the entire study population, as well as to generate hypotheses for future research (Cui et al. 2002). Finally, for the study of oncology, subgroup analyses are important to identify patients at increased risk for severe toxicity of the prescribed treatments. Subgroup analyses would likely be considered for important Tier I events.

When reporting results within subgroups, transparency is key for appropriate interpretation of results. Details on the number of subgroups assessed (not just reported), whether subgroups were determined pre- or post-hoc, multiplicity adjustments were applied, stratified randomization was used, or heterogeneity was assessed through interaction tests should be clearly described (Lagakos 2006; Wang et al. 2007). For multiplicity, details as to whether adjusted or unadjusted *p*-values are presented or simultaneous or unadjusted confidence or credible intervals should be clearly described. However, the regulatory guidance appears to prefer presenting unadjusted *p*-values and intervals for subgroup analyses as they are "investigations [that] serve as an indicator for further exploration" (CHMP 2014). Even though power tends to be low for tests of interaction, many authors suggest that heterogeneity of treatment effects should always be evaluated, and regulatory guidance encourages reporting estimates and confidence intervals for these interaction tests (Pocock et al. 2002, Lagakos 2006, CHMP 2014). Further, the literature highlights that the presence and the size of interaction depend on the choice of the measure of divergence between the treatment groups (CHMP 2014; Chuang-Stein et al. 2014). The measures used to determine heterogeneity should be prespecified and clearly documented.

Table 8.4 summarizes the incidence of rash/desquamation from two studies of two doses of imatinib (400 and 800 mg) for the treatment of unresectable or metastatic gastrointestinal stromal tumors (GIST); rash/desquamation was selected due to the large treatment effect between the two doses. The results in Table 8.4 are simulated using summary results from the January 2015 imatinib drug label and a meta-analysis of the two clinical trials (MetaGIST 2010; Novartis Pharmaceutical Corporation 2015). Figure 8.3 contains a summary of rash/desquamation within subgroups for the EU-AUS trial reported in Table 8.4. The left panel presents a forest plot that summarizes overall and subgroup estimates and unadjusted 95% confidence

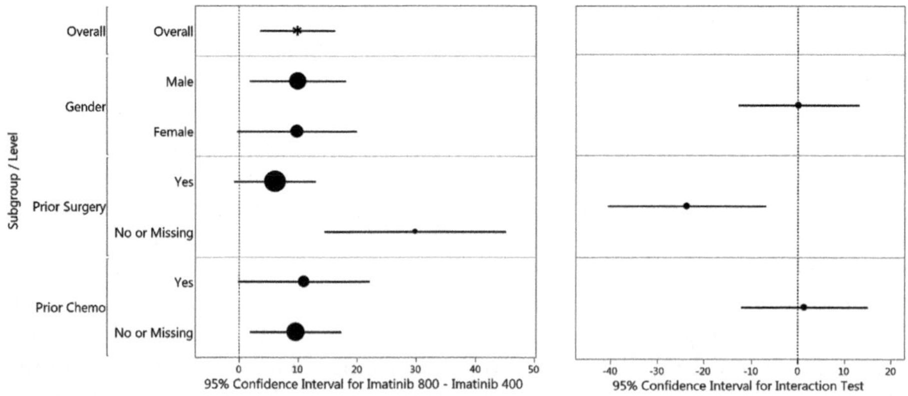

FIGURE 8.3
Subgroup analysis of rash/desquamation from EU-AUS GIST Trial. Unadjusted 95% confidence intervals are based on the risk difference of imatinib 800mg minus imatinib 400mg using a normal approximation. Interaction tests are based on unadjusted 95% confidence intervals for the difference in treatment effects between the two subgroup levels (level 1 minus level 2). Bubble area is proportional to the total number of patients within each subgroup level.

TABLE 8.4

Simulated Table of Rash/Desquamation from a Meta-Analysis of Two Doses of Imatinib for the Treatment of Unresectable or Metastatic GISTs

	EU-AUS ($N = 946$)		US-CAN ($N = 694$)	
	Imatinib (400 mg)	**Imatinib (800 mg)**	**Imatinib (400 mg)**	**Imatinib (800 mg)**
Overall	193/473 (40.8)	240/473 (50.7)	119/345 (34.5)	169/349 (48.4)
Male	120/297 (40.4)	139/276 (50.4)	72/171 (42.1)	98/205 (47.8)
Female	73/176 (41.5)	101/197 (51.3)	47/174 (27.0)	71/144 (49.3)
Prior surgery—yes	174/394 (44.2)	205/408 (50.2)	99/297 (33.3)	140/290 (48.3)
Prior surgery—no or missing	19/79 (24.1)	35/65 (53.8)	20/48 (41.7)	29/59 (49.2)
Prior chemo—yes	73/177 (41.2)	70/134 (52.2)	33/76 (43.4)	40/75 (53.3)
Prior chemo—no or missing	120/296 (40.5)	170/339 (50.1)	86/269 (32.0)	129/274 (47.1)

Values are a number of patients with rash/desquamation over the total number of patients and (%). The table is simulated using data of combined overall treatment arms from Table 12 of Novartis Pharmaceuticals Corporation (2015, Jan) and Table A1 of baseline demographic and clinical characteristics from Gastrointestinal Stromal Tumor Meta-Analysis Group (2010). The total incidences of rash/desquamation for the two trials from the drug label are 312/818 (38.1) and 409/822 (49.8) for Imatinib 400 and 800 mg, respectively.

intervals for the risk difference of imatinib 800 mg minus imatinib 400 mg using a normal approximation. Bubble area is proportional to the size of the subgroup level. On the basis of recommendations from the CHMP (2014), interaction tests are summarized using a forest plot in the right panel and are based on unadjusted 95% confidence intervals for the difference in treatment effects between the two subgroup levels (level 1 minus level 2, e.g., male effect minus female effect). With sufficient space, a dot plot could be added to Figure 8.3 to summarize the incidence rates of rash/desquamation to complete a safety triptych.

8.4.3 Meta-Analysis

While FDR can limit false-positives without overly sacrificing power, the rarity of many safety endpoints will require a meta-analysis of multiple studies for sufficient power to generate meaningful inference for the safety population, as well as more precise estimates of the treatment response within various subgroups (Crowe et al. 2009; Berlin et al. 2012, Chuang-Stein et al. 2014). Meta-analyses should be preplanned and assess the heterogeneity and poolability of the included clinical trials, and not simply reflect a naïve grouping of patients from multiple studies, ignoring the variability in treatment effects between studies. As an additional benefit, the availability of multiple trials allows the analyst to assess the consistency of response within a particular subgroup from one study to the next (i.e., replication). As Li and coauthors point out, it is possible to observe negative results (even significantly so) within at least one subgroup when the result is known to be homogeneous among all subgroups (Li et al. 2007). Chuang-Stein et al. (2014) provide details and recommendations for fixed and random effects models for meta-analyses of safety endpoints.

In general, the overall treatment effect θ, assuming a fixed effects meta-analysis model for a total of s studies, can be estimated using $\hat{\theta} = \sum_{h=1}^{s} \hat{\theta}_h w_h \Big/ \sum_{h=1}^{s} w_h$, where $\hat{\theta}_h$ is the estimated treatment effect and w_h is the weight for the hth study (Whitehead 2002). For a binary outcome with the Mantel–Haenszel weights $w_h = \dfrac{n_{\text{ht}} n_{\text{hc}}}{n_h}$ and difference in proportions between treatment t and control c defined as $\hat{\theta}_h = \hat{p}_{\text{ht}} - \hat{p}_{\text{hc}}$ for the hth study, a 95% confidence interval for the overall difference in proportions is $\hat{\theta} \pm 1.96 \sqrt{\hat{\theta}\left(\sum_{h=1}^{s} U_h\right) + \left(\sum_{h=1}^{s} V_h\right) \Big/ \left(\sum_{h=1}^{s} \dfrac{n_{\text{ht}} n_{\text{hc}}}{n_h}\right)^2}$, where $U_h = \dfrac{n_{\text{ht}}^2 x_{\text{hc}} - n_{\text{hc}}^2 x_{\text{ht}} + n_{\text{ht}} n_{\text{hc}} (n_{\text{hc}} - n_{\text{ht}})/2}{n_h^2}$, $V_h = \dfrac{x_{\text{ht}} (n_{\text{hc}} - x_{\text{hc}}) + x_{\text{hc}} (n_{\text{ht}} - x_{\text{ht}})}{2n_h}$, and x_{ht} x_{hc} are the number of successes in the hth study for the treatment and control groups, respectively (Chuang-Stein et al. 2014).

Figure 8.4 summarizes unadjusted 95% confidence intervals for rash/desquamation for the EU-AUS and US-CAN trials for the risk difference of imatinib 800 mg minus imatinib 400 mg using a normal approximation. The Overall Naïve result is based on the grouping of the data for the two trials (312/818 and 409/822 for Imatinib 400 and 800 mg, respectively) and computing an unadjusted 95% confidence interval for the risk difference using a normal approximation. The overall meta-analysis result uses the abovementioned formulas from Chuang-Stein et al. (2014). While there is little difference visually between the two intervals using data from both trials, the confidence interval for the overall meta-analysis is expected to be wider since it accounts for the variability in treatment effects between studies. This display summarizes the overall results, but also allows the reader to assess the variability of findings for the individual trials. As expected, the estimate of the overall meta-analysis is between the two trials, and the confidence interval is narrower. As in Figure 8.3, a second forest plot could be provided to summarize the heterogeneity of the included clinical trials. Finally, it is important to note that any meta-analysis methods utilized should summarize the results of all appropriate oncology studies to avoid biased conclusions—this includes trials where treatment arms may experience no events or single-arm (See Tian et al. 2009, as an example).

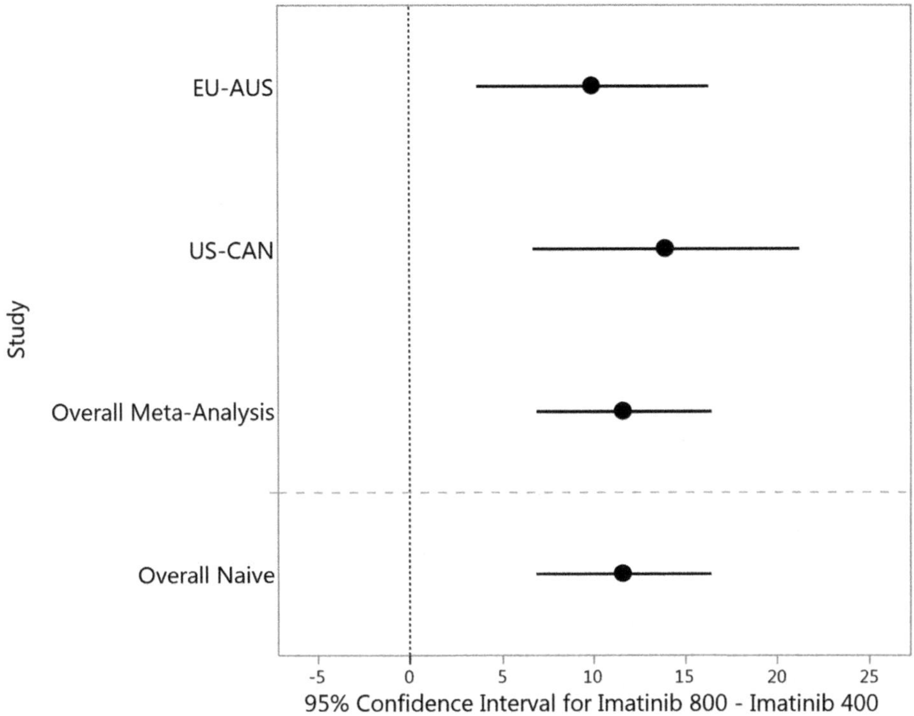

FIGURE 8.4
Meta-analysis of rash/desquamation from EU-AUS and US-CAN GIST trials. Unadjusted 95% confidence intervals for rash/desquamation for the EU-AUS and US-CAN trials are based on the risk difference of imatinib 800 mg minus imatinib 400 mg using a normal approximation. The overall Naïve results are based on the grouping of the data for the two trials (312/818 and 409/822 for matinib 400 and 800 mg, respectively) and computing an unadjusted 95% confidence interval for the risk difference using a normal approximation. The overall meta-analysis result use the formulas from Chuang-Stein et al. (2014).

8.4.4 Other Safety Endpoints

Numerous other data are collected in clinical trials, all of which can indicate a safety concern. Here, we focus on laboratory measurements, though any continuously reported outcomes can utilize the methods mentioned here. As described in Section 8.4.1, occurrences of clinically relevant changes in other safety endpoints are often reported as AEs. Alternatively, measures can be dichotomized according to one or more clinically meaningful thresholds (e.g., lab measures above or below the upper or lower limits of normal, respectively). While dichotomizing continuous or multilevel outcomes results in a loss of information, all of the abovementioned methodologies for binary outcomes would apply (Senn 2003; Federov et al. 2009). One important point raised in Chuang-Stein (1995) is the recommendation to use central laboratories for the consistency in laboratory findings across all sites. In general, similar methods of collection and evaluation should apply to all data, particularly those with subjective interpretations. Event adjudication for death and disease progression to ascertain whether patients met the criteria for primary endpoints follows similar thinking (Crowe et al. 2009).

Analyses of laboratory measurements or other safety outcomes may not uncover any noticeable differences between the treatment arms. This should not be too surprising since clinical trials are not powered to detect differences among the many safety outcomes that are measured. However, screening for unusual changes in laboratory measurements within a patient may help uncover individuals who are at risk for a more serious safety outcome. Given the number of endpoints and the different ways in which to summarize potential risk, graphics makes it straightforward to identify patients experiencing significant changes, and highlights potential trends between the treatment groups. In oncology, shift tables are typically used to identify changes in toxicity grade from baseline by treatment arm and cycle. Alternatively, shift plots summarize baseline values versus on-study (overall or by cycle) averages, minimums, or maximums, making it straightforward to identify patients with noticeable changes during treatment. Further, the presence of a majority of the points on the left or right side of the diagonal reference line indicates an increase or decrease of the endpoint, respectively, for a particular treatment arm, or the entire study population. Figure 8.5 presents a shift plot for ALT normalized by the upper limit of normal (ULN) for a simulated two-arm trial of 100 patients. The values of the x- and y-axes indicate log2 multipliers of the ULN; every unit implies a doubling of the observed ALT result compared to the ULN. Depending on the endpoint, other clinically relevant transformations (including no transformation) could be considered. On the basis of the applied transformation, appropriate reference lines can be added to identify patients who have crossed clinically relevant thresholds. Shift plots can be further enhanced by fitting regression lines to emphasize any trends within and between the treatments, or points can be colored according to important changes in toxicity grade. Shift plots can also be used to summarize differences in toxicity grade between baseline and the treatment phase, employing symbol size to indicate the frequency of patients at a particular (X,Y) coordinate, and utilizing bubble transparency or open rings (as in Figure 8.1) so that all treatments arms are visible within the same plot.

Similarly, waterfall plots provide a graphical summary of change from baseline in measurements for all patients (Chuang-Stein et al. 2001). Figure 8.6 presents the change from baseline in an on-study average for ALT for 100 patients for a simulated two-arm trial of 100 patients. The plot clearly communicates that ALT increased for most patients and many of the largest changes occurred in patients on the experimental therapy. Reference lines can be added to identify important clinically relevant changes; p-values from

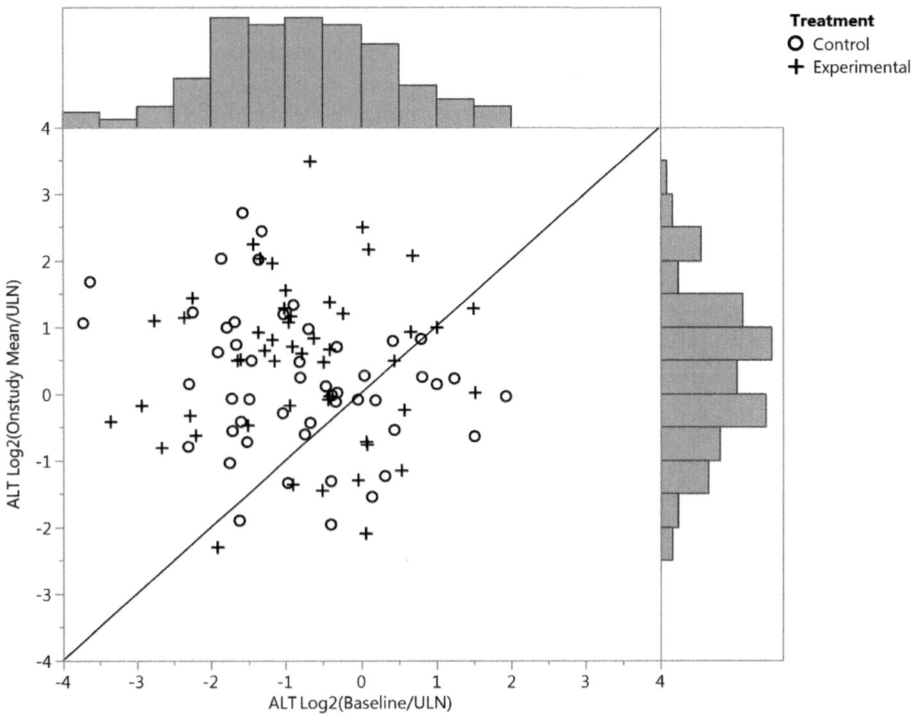

FIGURE 8.5
Shift plot of normalized ALT. Simulated values for normalized baseline and on-study average ALT for 100 patients randomized 1:1 to a control or experimental treatment. Diagonal reference line indicates no change between baseline and on-study mean ALT.

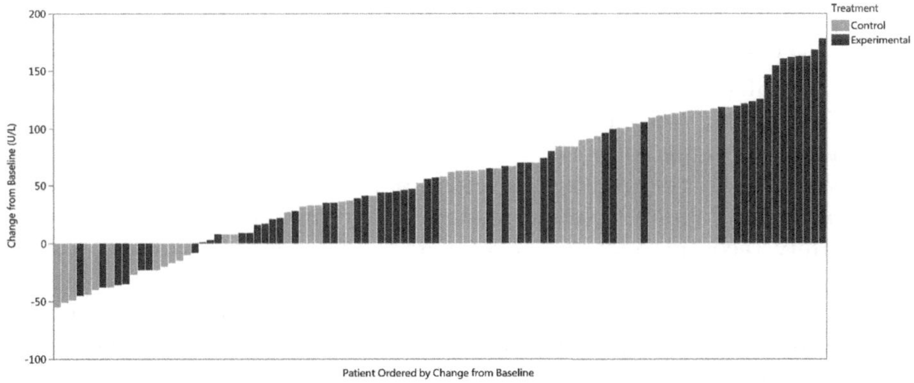

FIGURE 8.6
Waterfall plot of change from baseline for ALT. Simulated values for change from baseline of on-study average ALT for 100 patients randomized 1:1 to a control or experimental treatment.

Wilcoxon rank sum tests or randomization-based nonparametric analysis of covariance can be used to determine whether differences exist between treatments under minimal assumptions (Koch et al. 1993; Zink et al. 2017). In situations where the clinical interpretation of change from baseline on the observed measurement scale is unclear, percentage change from baseline can be used to present changes relative to each patients' baseline value, or the changes in NCI-CTCAE toxicity grades from baseline can be presented.

We summarized our recommendations for reporting safety in clinical trials of oncology, with a primary focus on AEs; sensitivity analyses can be performed on events that are more severe (NCI-CTCAE grades 3 and above), or are related to study medication in some way (ADRs). Due to limitations of available data, most of our discussion focused on the proportion of subjects experiencing a particular AE, without consideration for the length of time a patient was on the trial. Given the likelihood for death, disease progression, or dropout for patients in clinical trials of oncology, methodologies that account for patient exposure such as the exposure-adjusted incidence rate or time-to-first event would provide important sensitivity analyses (Liu et al. 2006; Collett 2015; Zhou et al. 2015). Similarly, analyses that account for the recurrence of events can and should be considered (Koch et al. 1993, Zhou et al. 2015). Koch et al. (1993) provide details for the meta-analysis of exposure-adjusted incidence or multiple events. The EMA highlights the importance of differential exposure between patient arms in Section 8.2 of their guidance document and stresses the need for analysis and presentation methods that consider the effect of time (EMA 2016). Presenting results by time and cycle as suggested at the end of Section 8.4.1 is an important first step. Zhou et al. (2015) raise an important point that extremely rare events should be analyzed using exact methods. Given the rarity of many individual events, an alternative strategy to identify safety signals is to analyze groups of terms that describe a particular medical condition using standardized MedDRA queries (SMQs) (Mozzicato 2007).

We have barely scratched the surface for the reporting of safety in oncology trials. Due to space considerations, we have neglected mentioning other important safety endpoints including the monitoring of ECG, as well as the analysis of patient-reported outcomes (PRO) to assess the tolerability of study treatments (the latter of which would utilize NCI's PRO-CTCAE grades). However, many of the analysis considerations described here would apply to these other endpoints. Of course, readers should first familiarize themselves with safety recommendations of regulatory agencies by reviewing appropriate guidance documents (e.g., EMA 2016). Readers interested in greater detail on the analysis and reporting of safety outcomes can explore recent texts by Jiang and Xia (2014) or Gould (2015), or revisit Gilbert (1993). Those interested in graphical presentations of safety data can review Chuang-Stein et al. (2001), Amit et al. (2008), Krause and O'Connell (2012), Duke et al. (2005), or Matange (2016).

8.5 Conclusions

There has been an increased interest in the systematic monitoring of safety for a compound throughout the drug development life cycle. While methods are available to monitor the safety of novel therapies in early oncology drug development, many challenges still remain. For example, it is often extremely difficult to assess the causality of AEs in relation to the investigational drug due to the severity of symptoms of the underlying disease, the toxicity from other concurrent therapies, and the frequent use of non-randomized study designs. Further, in randomized phase II and phase III studies, safety is considered to be one of the components of the BR trade-off, a complex and comprehensive process that requires an independent group of experts (DMC) to protect the well-being of patients in ongoing trials. It is no understatement to say that all randomized trials in oncology should have an independent DMC, comprised of members with diverse clinical and statistical expertise, and aided in their decisions through the use of stringent statistical stopping boundaries. Any decisions to terminate the trial early needs to be based on the totality of available evidence, both in the current trial and other external evidence. Stopping early for unconvincing results can have serious consequences. It is critical that the DMC, principal investigators, executive committees, and sponsors all recognize the full public health implications of their recommendations and decisions.

Finally, even though the case studies and a majority of the discussion in this chapter focused on cytotoxic drugs, the information and recommendations can be applicable to targeted drugs and immune modulators. We recognize that different dosing regimens and modes of action of these pharmacological entities affect the toxicity and tolerability profiles in different ways. Conventional cytotoxic drugs are typically given at weekly intervals and are characterized by major acute but transient toxicity, followed by recovery period prior to the next treatment cycle. For this reason, safety parameters (e.g., AEs and labs related to myelosuppression) in such trials are often analyzed and presented by the treatment cycle. Thus, the safety profile of cytotoxic drugs presents different challenges compared with targeted drugs or immune modulators that are administered continuously, either until disease progression or for a limited treatment period. For example, the main difference in the safety profile of immunotherapeutics is that these treatments seek to fight cancer by enhancing the immune system, often leading to unwanted autoimmune complications. Such AEs can appear early after a single treatment or perhaps even 20 or more weeks after the first dose. When monitoring and analyzing safety data, the specific characteristics of the underlying treatments should be taken into account when defining an appropriate analysis strategy.

References

Amit O, Heiberger RM, and Lane PW. Graphical approaches to the analysis of safety data from clinical trials. *Pharmaceutical Statistics* 7 (2008): 20–35.

Antonijevic Z, Gallo P, Chuang-Stein C, et al. Views on emerging issues pertaining to data monitoring committees for adaptive trials. *Therapeutic Innovation & Regulatory Science* 47(4) (2013): 495–502.

Benjamini Y and Hochberg Y. Controlling the false discovery rate: a practical and powerful approach to multiple testing. *Journal of the Royal Statistical Society B* 57 (1995): 289–300.

Benjamini Y and Yekutieli D. False discovery rate-adjusted multiple confidence intervals for selected parameters. *Journal of the American Statistical Association* 100 (2005): 71–81.

Berlin JA, Crowe BJ, Whalen E, et al. Meta-analysis of clinical trial safety data in a drug development program: answers to frequently asked questions. *Clinical Trials* 10 (2012): 20–31.

Berry DA. Adaptive clinical trials in oncology. *Nature Reviews Clinical Oncology* 9 (2012): 199–207.

Berry S, Carlin B, Lee JJ, and Muller P. *Bayesian Adaptive Methods for Clinical Trials.* CRC Press, Boca Raton (2011).

Brada M, Ashley S, Dowe A, et al. Neoadjuvant phase II multicentre study of new agents in patients with malignant glioma after minimal surgery. Report of a cohort of 187 patients treated with temozolomide. *Annals of Oncology* 16(6) (2005): 942–949.

Brown EG, Wood L, and Wood S. The medical dictionary for regulatory activities (MedDRA). *Drug Safety* 20 (1999): 109–117.

Bryant J and Day R. Incorporating toxicity considerations into the design of two-stage phase II clinical trials. *Biometrics* 51 (1995): 1372–1383.

Chen Y and Smith B. Adaptive group sequential designs for phase II clinical trials: a Bayesian decision theoretic approach. *Statistics in Medicine* 28 (2009): 3347–3362.

Chuang-Stein C, Ii Y, Kawai N, et al. Detecting safety signals in subgroups. In: Jiang Q & Xia HA, eds. *Quantitative Evaluation of Safety in Drug Development: Design, Analysis and Reporting.* Boca Raton, FL: CRC Press (2014).

Chuang-Stein C, Le V, and Chen W. Recent advancements in the analysis and presentation of safety data. *Drug Information Journal* 35 (2001): 377–397.

Chuang-Stein C. Points for consideration in the collection and analysis of safety data. *Drug Information Journal* 29 (1995): 37–44.

Collett D. *Modelling Survival Data in Medical Research.* (3rd ed.). CRC Press, Boca Raton, FL (2015).

Committee for Medicinal Products for Human Use (CHMP). Guideline on the investigation of subgroups in confirmatory clinical trials (draft). European Medicines Agency. Available at: http://www.ema.europa.eu/docs/en_GB/document_library/Scientific_guideline/2014/02/WC500160523.pdf (2014).

Conaway MR and Petroni GR. Designs for phase II trials allowing for trade-off between response and toxicity. *Biometrics* 52 (1996): 1375–1386.

Conaway MR and Petroni GR. Bivariate sequential designs for phase II trials. *Biometrics* 51 (1995): 656–664.

Crowe BJ, Xia HA, Berlin JA, et.al. Recommendations for safety planning, data collection, evaluation and reporting during drug, biologic and vaccine development: a report of the safety planning, evaluation, and reporting team. *Clinical Trials* 6 (2009): 430–440.

Cui L, Hung HMJ, Wang SJ, Tsong Y. Issues related to subgroup analysis in clinical trials. *Journal of Biopharmaceutical Statistics.* 12(3) (2002): 347–358.

Dixon D, Freedman R, Herson J, et al. Guidelines for data and safety monitoring for clinical trials not requiring traditional data monitoring committees. *Clinical Trials* 3 (2006): 314–319.

Duke SP, Bancken F, Crowe B, et al. Seeing is believing: good graphic design principles for medical research. *Statistics in Medicine* 34 (2005): 3040–3059.

Ellenberg SS, Fleming TR, and DeMets DL. *Data Monitoring Committees in Clinical Trials: A Practical Perspective.* John Wiley & Sons, (2002).

Elter T, Borchmann P, Schulz H, et al. Fludarabine in combination with alemtuzumab is effective and feasible in patients with relapsed or refractory B-cell chronic lymphocytic leukemia: results of a phase II trial. *Journal of Clinical Oncology* 23(28) (2005): 7024–7031.

European Medicines Agency (2016). Draft guideline on the evaluation of anticancer medicinal products in man.

European Medicines Agency (2016). Guideline on the scientific application and the practical arrangements necessary to implement the procedure for accelerated assessment pursuant to Article 14(9) of Regulation (EC) No 726/2004.

FDA (2006). *Guidance for Clinical Trial Sponsors: Establishment and Operation of Clinical Trial Data Monitoring Committees.*

FDA (2010). Food and Drug Administration. Guidance for Industry: Adaptive Design Clinical Trials for Drugs and Biologics Draft Guidance.

FDA (2014). Guidance for Industry on Expedited Programs for Serious Conditions – Drugs and Biologics.

FDA (2015). Draft Guidance for Industry on Safety Assessment for IND Safety Reporting.

Federov V, Mannino F, and Zhang R. Consequences of dichotomization. *Pharmaceutical Statistics* 8 (2009): 50–61.

Gallo P. Confidentiality and trial integrity issues for adaptive trials. *Drug Information Journal* 40 (2006a): 445–450.

Gallo P. Operational challenges in adaptive design implementation. *Pharmaceutical Statistics* 5 (2006b): 119–124.

Gandara D, Crowley J, Livingston R, et al. Evaluation of cisplatin in metastatic non-small cell lung cancer: a phase III study of the southwest oncology group. *Journal of Clinical Oncology* 11 (1993): 873–878.

Gastrointestinal Stromal Tumor Meta-Analysis Group (MetaGIST). Comparison of two doses of imatinib for the treatment of unresectable or metastatic gastrointestinal stromal tumors: A meta-analysis of 1,640 patients. *Journal of Clinical Oncology* 28 (2010): 1247–1253.

Geller NL, Follmann DF, Leifer ES, et al. Design of early trials in peripheral blood stem cell transplantation: a hybrid frequentist-Bayesian approach. In: Geller NL, ed. *Advances in Clinical Trial Biostatistics.* New York and Basel: Marcel Dekker (2005): 40–52.

George S, Freidlin B, and Korn E. Strength of accumulated evidence and data monitoring committee decision making. *Statistics in Medicine* 23 (2004): 2659–2672.

George S and Green M. Controversies in the early reporting of a clinical trial in early breast cancer. In: DeMets D, Furberg C, and Friedman L, eds. *Data Monitoring in Clinical Trials: A Case Studies Approach.* Springer (2006): 346–359.

Gibson MK, Catalano PJ, Kleinberg L, et al. (eds). E2205: a phase II study to measure response rate and toxicity of neoadjuvant chemoradiotherapy (CRT) with oxaliplatin (OX) and infusional 5-fluorouracil (5-FU) plus cetuximab (C) followed by postoperative docetaxel (DT) and C in patients with operable adenocarcinoma of the esophagus (abstr 4064). ASCO Annual Meeting, Chicago, IL, June 4–8 (2010) *Journal of Clinical Oncology* 28(15s) (2010): 4064. (suppl; abstr 4064).

Gilbert GS, ed. *Drug Safety Assessment in Clinical Trials.* Marcel Dekker, New York, NY: (1993).

Gould AL, ed. *Statistical Methods for Evaluating Safety in Medical Product Development.* John Wiley & Sons Ltd, Chichester, UK (2015).

Green S, Benedetti J, and Crowley J. *Clinical Trials in Oncology.* Chapman & Hall/ CRC (2003).

Haura EB, Ricart AD, Larson TG, et al. Phase II study of PD-0325901, anoral MEK inhibitor, in previously treated patients with advanced non-small cell lung cancer. *Clinical Cancer Research.* 16(8) (2010): 2450–2457.

Herson, J. Coordinating data monitoring committees and adaptive clinical trial designs. *Drug Information Journal* 42 (2008): 297–301.

Herson, J. Data and Safety Monitoring Committees in Clinical Trials. Boca Raton: Chapman & Hall/CRC Press (2009).

International Conference on Harmonisation. Guideline E2A: Clinical Safety Data Management: Definitions and Standards for Expedited Reporting. Available at: http://www.ich.org/fileadmin/Public_Web_Site/ICH_Products/Guidelines/Efficacy/E2A/Step4/E2A_Guideline.pdf (1994).

Ivanova A, Qaqish BF, and Schell MJ. Continuous toxicity monitoring in phase II trials in oncology. *Biometrics* 61 (2005): 540–546.

Ivanova A, Deal AM. Two-stage design for phase II oncology trials with relaxed futility stopping. *Statistics and its interface* 9(1) (2016): 93–98.

Jennison C and Turnbull B. *Group Sequential Methods, Applications to Clinical Trials.* Chapman & Hall/ CRC (2000).

Jiang Q and He W. eds. *Benefit-Risk Assessment Methods in Medical Product Development.* CRC Press, Boca Raton, FL (2016).

Jiang Q and Xia HA. eds. *Quantitative Evaluation of Safety in Drug Development: Design, Analysis and Reporting.* CRC Press, Boca Raton, FL (2014).

Jin W, Riley RM, Wolfinger RD, et al. The contributions of sex, genotype and age to transcriptional variance in Drosophila melanogaster. *Nature Genetics* 29 (2001): 389–395.

Kantarjian H, Shah NP, Hochhaus A, et.al. Dasatinib versus imatinib in newly diagnosed chronic-phase chronic myeloid leukemia. *New England Journal of Medicine* 362 (2010): 2260–2270.

Koch GG, Schmid JE, Begun JM, et.al. Meta-analysis of drug safety data. In: Gilbert GS, ed. *Drug Safety Assessment in Clinical Trials.* New York, NY: Marcel Dekker (1993).

Krause A and O'Connell M, eds. *A Picture is Worth a Thousand Tables: Graphics in Life Sciences.* Springer, New York, NY (2012).

Krug LM, Miller VA, Patel J, et al. Randomized phase II study of weekly docetaxel plus trastuzumab versus weekly paclitaxel plus trastuzumab in patients with previously untreated advanced nonsmall cell lung carcinoma. *Cancer* 104(10) (2005): 2149–2155.

Lagakos S. The challenge of subgroup analyses: Reporting without distorting. *New England Journal of Medicine* 354 (2006): 1667–1669.

Lewis R and Berry D. Group sequential clinical trials: a classical evaluation of bayesian decision-theoretic designs. *JASA* 89(428) (1994): 1528–1534.

Lewis S and Clarke M. Forest plots: trying to see the wood and the trees. *British Medical Journal* 322 (2001): 1479–1480.

Li Z, Chuang-Stein C, and Hoseyni C. The probability of observing negative subgroup results when the treatment effect Is positive and homogeneous across all subgroups. *Drug Information Journal* 41 (2007): 47–56.

Liu GF, Wang J, Liu K, et al. Confidence intervals for an exposure adjusted incidence rate difference with applications to clinical trials. *Statistics in Medicine* 25 (2006): 1275–1286.

Matange S. *Clinical Graphs Using SAS*. SAS Institute Inc, Cary, NC (2016).

Mehrotra DV and Adewale AJ. Flagging clinical adverse experiences: reducing false discoveries without materially compromising power for detecting true signals. *Statistics in Medicine* 31 (2012): 1918–1930.

Montori V, Devereaux P, Adhikari N, et al. Randomized trials stopped early for benefit: a systematic review. *JAMA* 204(17) 2005: 2203–2209.

Mozzicato P. Standardised MedDRA queries: their role in signal detection. *Drug Safety* 30 (2007): 617–619.

Novartis Pharmaceuticals Corporation. Prescribing Information for Gleevec (imatinib mesylate) tablets for oral use. (2015): Jan Available at: http://www.pharma.us.novartis.com/product/pi/pdf/gleevec_tabs.pdf.

O'Brien PC and Fleming TR. A multiple testing procedure for clinical trials. *Biometrics* 35 (1979): 549–556.

Penson RT, Dizon DS, Cannistra SA, et al. Phase II study of carboplatin, paclitaxel, and bevacizumab with maintenance bevacizumab as first-line chemotherapy for advanced mullerian tumors. *Journal of Clinical Oncology* 28(1) (2010): 154–159.

Pocock SJ, Assmann SE, Enos LE, et al. Subgroup analysis, covariate adjustment and baseline comparisons in clinical trial reporting: current practice and problems. *Statistics in Medicine* 21 (2002): 2917–2930.

Pocock SJ. Group sequential methods in the design and analysis of clinical trials. *Biometrika* 64 (1977): 191–199.

Pocock SJ. When (not) to stop a clinical trial for benefit. *JAMA* 294 (2005): 2228–2230.

Quan H, Mingyu L, Chen J, et.al. Assessment of consistency of treatment effects in multiregional clinical trials. *Drug Information Journal* 44 (2010): 617–632.

Reiner E, Paoletti X, and O'Quigley J. Operating characteristics of the standard phase I clinical trial design. *Computational Statistics & Data Analysis* 30 (1999): 303–315.

Ross HJ, Blumenschein GR Jr, Aisner J, et al. Randomized phase II multicenter trial of two schedules of lapatinib as first- or second-line monotherapy in patients with advanced or metastatic non-small cell lung cancer. *Clinical Cancer Research* 16(6) (2010): 1938–1949.

Samon S, Crowley J, Balcerzak S, et al. Interferon versus interferon plus prednisone remission maintenance therapy for multiple myeloma: a southwest oncology group study, *Journal of Clinical Oncology* 16 (1998): 890–896.

Senn S. Disappointing dichotomies. *Pharmaceutical Statistics* 2 (2003): 239–240.

Simon R. Optimal two-stage designs for phase II clinical trials. *Controlled Clinical Trials* 10 (1989): 1–10.

Song, G and Ivanova, A. Frequentist enrollment and stopping rules for managing toxicity requiring long follow-up in Phase II oncology trials. *Journal of Biopharmaceutical Statistics* 25(6) (2015): 1206–1214.

Thall P. Some geometric methods for constructing decision criteria based on two-dimensional parameters. *Journal of Statistical Planning and Inference* 138 (2008): 516–527.

Thall PF and Sung HG. Some extensions and applications of a Bayesian strategy for monitoring multiple outcomes in clinical trials. *Statistics in Medicine* 17 (1998): 1563–1580.

Thall PF and Cheng SC. Treatment comparisons based on two-dimensional safety and efficacy alternatives in oncology trials. *Biometrics* 55 (1999): 746–753.

Thall PF, Simon RM, and Estey EH. Bayesian sequential monitoring designs for single-arm clinical trials with multiple outcomes. *Statistics in Medicine* 14 (1995): 357–379.

Thall PF, Simon RM, and Estey EH. New statistical strategy for monitoring safety and efficacy in for single-arm clinical trials. *Journal of Clinical Oncology* 14 (1996): 296–303.

Tian L, Cai T, Pfeffer MA, et al. Exact and efficient inference procedure for meta-analysis and its application to the analysis of independent 2x2 tables with all available data but without artificial continuity correction. *Biostatistics* 10 (2009): 275–281.

Trotta F, Apolone G, Garattini S, et al. Stopping a trial early in oncology: for patients or for industry? *Annals of Oncology* 19(7) (2008): 1347–1353.

Wang R, Lagakos, SW, Ware JH, et.al. Statistics in medicine - Reporting of subgroup analyses in clinical trials. *New England Journal of Medicine* 357 (2007): 2189–2194.

Whitehead A. *Meta-Analysis of Controlled Clinical Trials.* John Wiley & Sons Ltd, Chichester, England (2002).

Zhou Y, Ke C, Jiang Q, et al. Choosing appropriate metrics to evaluate adverse events in safety evaluation. *Therapeutic Innovation and Regulatory Science* 49 (2015): 398–404.

Zink RC, Koch GG, Chung Y, et al. Advanced randomization-based methods in clinical trials. In: Dmitrienko A & Koch GG, eds. *Analysis of Clinical Trials Using SAS: A Practical Guide* (2nd ed.). Cary, NC: SAS Institute Inc. (2017).

Zink RC, Wolfinger RD, and Mann G. Summarizing the incidence of adverse events using volcano plots and time windows. *Clinical Trials* 10 (2013): 398–406.

9

Quality of Life

Diane Fairclough

Colorado School of Public Health

CONTENTS

9.1 Introduction

Therapies for cancer are typically evaluated on the basis of disease progression and survival and utilize endpoints that are physical or laboratory measures of response. Although these measures are often the primary endpoints, they do not reflect how the patient feels and functions in daily activities. Yet, these perceptions reflect whether or not the patient believes he or she has benefited from the treatment. The patient's perception of his or her wellbeing may be the most important health outcome [36]. More recently, trials have included endpoints that reflect the patient's perception of his or her wellbeing and satisfaction with therapy. This is likely to become more common with targeted therapies that are hoped to be less toxic.

The term "quality of life" (QOL) is used in a variety of ways. In this chapter, I will use it as a surrogate for measures of health-related quality of life (HRQoL) as well as other patient-reported outcomes such as health status and symptoms.

There are a number of statistical challenges associated with the use of QOL measures in oncology trials. The first is determining the role of the QOL assessments given that survival or disease progression is typically the primary endpoint. The second challenge is how the potential multiplicity of endpoints will be handled. This includes all primary and secondary endpoints as well as the multiplicity generated by the longitudinal assessments (multiple time points) on multiple scales (e.g., physical well-being, emotional well-being, or multiple symptoms). The final challenge is missing data due to morbidity and mortality, especially the latter. All these challenges are discussed in this chapter.

9.2 QOL as an Endpoint in Cancer Trials

Given that most cancer clinical trials are designed to identify new drugs or combinations that improve survival, the role of QOL measures is often questioned. There are, however, important roles for QOL measures depending on the setting and the nature of the treatments. At the two extremes of the cancer trajectory, adjuvant therapy and stage IV disease, most experimental treatments relative to the active control intervention have minimal, if any, impact on survival. In the context of adjuvant therapy, any side effects such as fatigue or bone pain is likely to impact compliance, and thus, the potential benefits of one treatment over the other. At the other extreme, therapies for advanced stage disease typically have a modest impact on survival and their benefits are thus typically palliative as measured by QOL endpoints.

Even in the evaluation of interventions likely to change survival, there are lessons to be learned from QOL outcomes. Sometimes clinical investigators assume that a change in a biomedical outcome will also improve the patient's QOL. While in many cases this may be true, sometimes, surprising results are obtained when the patient is asked directly. One classic example of this occurred with a study by Sugarbaker et al. [37] comparing two therapeutic approaches for soft tissue sarcoma—limb-sparing surgery followed by radiation versus full amputation. The investigators hypothesized that "sparing a limb, as opposed to amputating it, offers a quality-of-life advantage." Most would have agreed with this conjecture. But the trial results did not confirm the expectations; subjects receiving the limb-sparing procedures reported limitations in mobility and sexual functioning. These observations were confirmed with physical assessments of mobility and endocrine function. As a result of these studies, radiation therapy was modified and physical rehabilitation was added to the limb-sparing therapeutic approach [16]. With our new generation of targeted therapies, we believe they will be less toxic and thus result in improved QOL; however, this needs to be demonstrated.

An example where there were no survival differences and the QOL measures were critical in determining the value of the intervention is a trial in metastatic prostate cancer that evaluated the effects of flutamide versus placebo. There were no statistically significant differences in survival. However, the patient in the flutamide arm experienced more symptoms of diarrhea at 3 months and poorer emotional functioning at 3 and 6 months [28].

Identifying the role of QOL as an endpoint is a critical step in the design of a trial. Roles differ from aims and could range from the primary measure that demonstrates efficacy or safety in a registration trial to solely exploratory for the purpose of hypothesis generation. The exact nature of the role will obviously guide the analysis plan, but will also determine the resources that will be employed to insure compliance with assessments.

9.3 Multiple Endpoints

It is well-known that performing multiple hypothesis tests and basing inference on unadjusted p-values increase the overall probability of false-positive results (Type-I errors). Multiple hypothesis tests in trials assessing HRQoL arises from three sources: 1) multiple HRQoL measures (scales or subscales), 2) repeated post-randomization assessments, and 3) multiple treatment arms. As a result, multiple testing is one of the major analytic challenges in these trials [21]. Not only does this create concerns about the type-I error, but reports containing large numbers of statistical tests generally result in a confusing picture of HRQoL that is hard to interpret.

Although widely used in the analysis of HRQoL in clinical trials [35], univariate tests of each HRQoL domain or scale and time point can seriously inflate the type-I (false-positive) error rate for the overall trial such that the researcher is unable to distinguish between the true and false differences. Post hoc adjustment is often infeasible because, at the end of the analysis, it is impossible to determine the number of tests performed.

So what are the options? The first is to limit hypothesis tests to a limited number of measures that have been prespecified in the trial design. The second is to consider summary measures or statistics across time or across subscales. And the third is to utilize multiple comparisons adjustments or gatekeeping strategies. Typically, we use a combination of all three approaches.

9.3.1 Summary Measures and Statistics

Two dimensions of measurement lend themselves to summary measures and statistics. The first is the multiple scales that measure the general and disease-specific domains of HRQoL and the second is the assessment over time. Developing composite measures from multiple scales is more controversial as it leads to endpoints that are a combination of different aspects of QOL that may or may not be impacted in the same direction. If all of the components are affected in the same direction and to a comparable extent, the composite is interpretable and clinically useful. However, if the components are affected in different directions, the use of the composite may miss the detection of treatment-related differences. Finally, if only one of the components drives the observed differences, the results may be misinterpreted as implying an impact on all the components [14].

Summary statistics across time are a very useful way of minimizing the impact of multiple comparisons procedures as well as facilitating the interpretation of results. Examples of summary statistics are area under the curve (AUC), an average of post-intervention measurements minus baseline, and slope. The choice depends on the trial design and usefulness to clinical practice. For example, if the intervention has a limited duration, two statistics might be proposed—one reflecting on the impact of treatment while on therapy and the other on post-therapy. Depending on the impact of the intervention on disease control and survival, either may be clinically useful. As an example, if a more toxic intervention has better disease control and equivalent post-intervention QOL, poor QOL during therapy could be used to provide patient education and thus improve compliance. When therapy does not have a defined (limited) duration (e.g., it is continued in the absence of disease progression), a summary measure such as the AUC may be useful.

There are also two approaches to summarizing longitudinal data. The first is to develop a strategy to compute a measure within each individual and then to perform univariate analysis on that measure. This sounds very attractive, but in practice, creating rules *a priori* that cover all contingencies is very difficult. A more practical approach is to select a method of analysis that addresses missing data as described later in Section 9.4 and then to compute summary statistics as linear combinations of the estimated parameters [11].

9.3.2 Multiple Comparisons Adjustments and Gatekeeping Strategies

There are numerous multiple comparison adjustment procedures. The most well-known and the most conservative is the Bonferroni adjustment, which divides alpha by the number of tests to be performed. Alternatives that are slightly less conservative include Holm's step-down procedure [19], Hochberg's step-up procedure [17], and the false discovery rate procedure. However, all of these procedures reduce the power to detect meaningful differences unless the trial is very large.

The critical trial decision is whether to control the type-I error solely at the level of the primary endpoints with no adjustments for secondary endpoints. Alternatives include controlling the type-I error for both primary and secondary endpoints. An innovative procedure not often used is the gatekeeping strategy. It requires a very clear specification of the roles of each of the outcomes (e.g., survival, disease progression, and QOL). In some settings, there is a prespecified sequence of testing families of hypotheses. Trial designs can include those with a single primary and multiple secondary endpoints (if the primary is nonsignificant, all other endpoints are irrelevant), multiple co-primary endpoints (significance of any of the primary endpoints is meaningful), and joint co-primary endpoints (tests of all primary endpoints need to be significant). In all of these designs, the two families of hypotheses are tested sequentially with the first family acting as a gatekeeper for the second family. Ideally, the gatekeeping strategy is based on a mechanistic model in which the first family consists of measures of a proximal effect of the intervention on outcomes and the second family consists of more distal outcomes. For example, the first family could consist of biological and physiological factors and the second could consist of measures of symptoms. Or the first family could consist of symptom status and the second family of measures of the perceived impact of those symptoms.

QOL endpoints typically are poorly integrated into clinical trials. However, a gatekeeping procedure with sequential families provides one strategy for better integration. As an illustration, consider a trial with hypotheses A, B, and C testing treatment differences in disease response, survival, and QOL. Let's assume hypothetically that the unadjusted (marginal) *p*-values are $p_A = 0.08$, $p_B = 0.02$, and $p_C = 0.03$ as indicated in Table 9.1. We will consider four scenarios (three of which consist of sequential families of hypotheses) to illustrate the methods. The closed-testing procedure proposed by Marcus [27] provides a theoretical basis for controlling the experiment-wise type-I error in a wide variety of settings. Dmitrienko et al. [8] present a formal way of displaying the procedure. The concepts are presented here; details are illustrated by Fairclough [11].

TABLE 9.1

Reported p-values for Multiple Hypotheses Using Gatekeeping Strategies

		Design 1	Design 2	Design 3	Design 4
Endpoint	**Unadjusted p-value**	**All Primary**	**Single Primary**	**Co-Primary**	**Joint Co-Primary**
A: Disease control	0.08	0.24	0.08	0.16	0.16
B: Survival	0.02	0.06	0.08	0.04	0.04
C: QOL	0.03	0.09	0.08	0.04	0.16
[0.5 ex]					

9.3.2.1 Design 1. All Primary with Bonferroni Corrections

If all three endpoints were considered primary endpoints and the Bonferroni procedure is used for the multiple comparisons adjustment, the null hypothesis for none of the comparisons would be rejected and the reported p-values would be 0.24, 0.06, and 0.09, respectively. In this scenario, the results for the Holms and Hochberg procedures would be qualitatively the same, though the p-values would differ.

9.3.2.2 Design 2. Single Primary Endpoint

In the second design, assume that disease control (H_A) was designated as the primary endpoint and both survival (H_B) and HRQoL (H_C) were designated as the secondary endpoints. The first family consists of H_A and the second family of H_B and H_C. In this design, if the null hypothesis for the primary endpoint (A) is not rejected, all of the secondary null hypotheses must be accepted. If we applied this design using the unadjusted p-values from the previous example, the adjusted p-values would be 0.08, 0.08, and 0.08. Thus, none of the three null hypotheses are rejected and the (adjusted) results are negative for all three endpoints.

9.3.2.3 Design 3. Co-Primary Endpoints

In the third design, disease control and survival (A and B) are the co-primary endpoints and QOL the secondary endpoint. If either hypothesis in the first family (H_A or H_B) is rejected, then the second family of hypotheses will be considered. The hypotheses in the first family are tested as if the Bonferroni procedure was applied to two endpoints. The adjusted p-values are 0.16 and 0.04. The adjusted p-value for the second family cannot be smaller than the smallest in the first family because the gatekeeping procedure requires that H_C cannot be rejected unless one of the hypotheses in the first family is rejected. Thus, $\tilde{p}_B = 0.04$. With design 3, we would reject the null hypotheses associated with one of the primary endpoints, survival, and for the secondary endpoint, QoL.

9.3.2.4 Design 4. Joint Co-Primary Endpoints

In the final design, disease control and survival are joint co-primary endpoints. This design differs from the previous as it requires both H_A and H_B to be rejected before considering the second family of hypotheses. The adjusted p-values for the first family of hypotheses are identical to those in Design 3. Because the gatekeeping procedure requires that H_C cannot be rejected unless both of the hypotheses in the first family are rejected, the adjusted p-value cannot be smaller than the largest in the first family; thus, $\tilde{p}_C = 0.16$. Thus, in design 4, only the survival hypotheses are rejected.

9.4 Missing Data

Patient-reported data missing due to morbidity or mortality is a common occurrence in oncology trials. These missing assessments are very rarely completely random, that is, unrelated to the current status of the individual at the time of the planned assessment (e.g., missing completely at random (MCAR)). Nor is missingness unrelated to the current status even after adjusting for previous data (e.g., missing at random (MAR) or patient characteristics measured at baseline). While there are formal tests of MCAR vs. MAR [23], there is no way to formally differentiate between MAR and missing not at random (MNAR) because we are missing the data that would be needed to exclude the possibility that missing data are mostly MNAR. It is possible to find evidence that data are not MAR, assuming a particular model [7,34,40], but the lack of evidence under a particular model does not confirm the data to be MAR. These issues are the basis for the recommendations to plan for a sensitivity analysis and the use of the term "sensitivity". It is the probable occurrence of nonrandom missing data (e.g.,MNAR) in a large proportion of patients and our inability to prove otherwise is a major challenge in the analysis and interpretation of QOL assessments in oncology trials.

9.4.1 Examples

The first example is a trial in advanced non–small cell lung cancer (NSCLC) [1]. Figure 9.1 illustrates the average trajectories as a function of the last observed assessment. If the missing data were MCAR, then the lines would overlap. The roughly fan-shaped trajectories suggest that the dropout (missingness) is associated with both the initial value and slope. A second example comes from a renal cell carcinoma trial [29]; the trajectories are nonlinear but also suggest that the dropout is related to the previously observed values and thus not MCAR (Figure 9.2). Additional analyses (described by

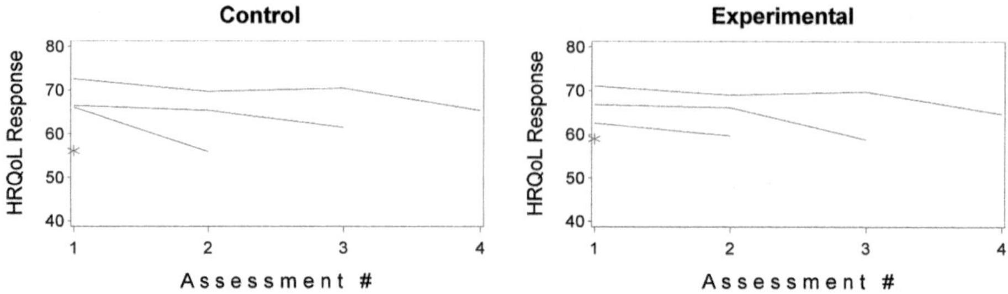

FIGURE 9.1
Average FACT-Lung TOI (a composite of physical, functional, and disease-specific symptoms) scores for the control (left) and experimental (right) arms stratified by the time of last assessment.

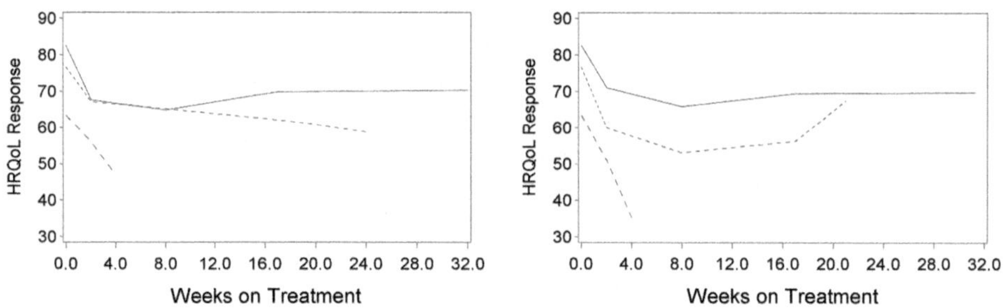

FIGURE 9.2
Average FACT-BRM TOI scores for control (left) and experimental (right) arms stratified by the time of last assessment. Patients with 25+ weeks of follow-up are represented by the solid line, those between 5 and 25 weeks of follow-up with the short dashed lines, and those with less than 5 weeks of follow-up with the long dashed lines.

Fairclough [11]) in conjunction with clinical expertise strongly suggest that the missing data is MNAR.

9.4.2 How Much Data Can be Missing?

There are no magic rules about how much missing data is acceptable in a clinical trial. The seriousness of the problem depends on the reasons for the missing data, the objectives of the study, and the intended use of the results. The tolerance in trials of adjuvant therapy will be low, whereas the tolerance for patients with metastatic disease will be much higher. When the proportion of missing assessments is very small (<5%), the potential bias or impact on power may be very minor. In some cases, 10%–20% missing data will have little or no effect on the results of the study. In other studies, 10%–20% may matter. As the proportion of the missing data increases to 30%–50%, the conclusions that one is willing to draw will be restricted.

9.4.3 Informative Missing Data Due to Dropout

9.4.3.1 *Methods to be Avoided*

Methods that assume the data to be MCAR, particularly those that do not utilize all the available data, will result in biased estimates of change in QOL over time and may result in biased comparisons of the treatment arms. Limiting the analysis to those who have completed all assessments (complete case analyses) is the most well-known example and is rarely used anymore. However, repeated univariate analyses of each endpoint at each time point is still frequently employed. As it does not utilize information from assessments at other time points, it assumes that assessments are MCAR and thus is biased in most oncology trials. Generalized estimating equations (GEEs) [18,32] also assume the data are MCAR. These methods have been extended using re-weighting techniques. These assume the "similarity" between subjects with data and subjects without data. This is typically not true in oncology trials.

9.4.3.2 *Recommended Approach*

In most oncology trials, missing data is associated with toxicity, disease progression, or death, and thus is likely to be non-ignorable (e.g., MNAR). Most experts recommend a likelihood-based approach using all available data supplemented by a sensitivity analysis [2,11,18]. The choice between growth curve mixed models [5] and repeated measures mixed models [20] will depend on the timing and the number of assessments. Trials with a limited number of assessments (2–5) that can be thought of as ordered categories (e.g., pre, early, late, and post therapy) and where all assessments can be uniquely classified are typically analyzed using a repeated measures model: $Y_i = X_i\beta + \epsilon_i$ for the i-th subject where the variance, Σ_i is unstructured. These trials are typical for interventions of limited duration. Trials with a larger number of assessments or where the timing of assessments becomes more varied over time are typically analyzed using the growth curve models that incorporate random effects: $Y_i = X_i\beta + Z_i d_i + \varepsilon_i$. The random effects, $Z_i d_i$, typically allow variation of the subject-specific intercepts and slope relative to the predicted trajectory. The variance is structured, $\Sigma_i = Z_i' D Z_i + \sigma^2 I$.

9.4.4 Sensitivity Analyses

In most oncology trials, non-ignorable missing data should be suspected. Determining the dropout mechanism would require knowledge about the data that is missing. These issues are the basis for the recommendations to plan for a sensitivity analysis and the use of the term "sensitivity."

There are a number of popular methods for sensitivity analyses. All require strong assumptions and are difficult to be prespecified prior to data collection. The common theme among them is that they attempt to convert the problem to one that is conditionally MAR. For example, the assumption underlying pattern mixture models is that the data are MAR within each pattern [11].

9.4.4.1 Mixture Models

The basic concept of mixture models is that the true distribution of the measures of HRQoL for the entire group of patients is a mixture of the distributions from each of the P groups of patients [24–26]. The distribution of the responses, Y_i, may differ across the P strata with different parameters, $\beta^{\{p\}}$, and variance, $\Sigma^{\{p\}}$.

$$Y_i \mid M^{\{p\}} \sim N\left(X_i\beta^{\{p\}}, \Sigma_i^{\{p\}}\right), p = 1,\ldots,P. \tag{9.1}$$

The complete data, $f(Y)$, is characterized as a mixture (weighted average) of the conditional distribution, $f(Y \mid M)$, over the distribution of dropout times, the patterns of missing data, or the random coefficients. The specific form of M distinguishes the various mixture models where M is either dropout time, T_i^D, the pattern of missing data, R_i, or a random coefficient, d_i.

$$\text{Pattern mixture } f\left(Y_i \mid R_i\right) \tag{9.2}$$

$$\text{Time-to-event mixture } f\left(Y_i \mid T_i^D\right) \tag{9.3}$$

$$\text{Random effects mixture } f\left(Y_i \mid d_i\right) \tag{9.4}$$

Pattern mixture models are a special case of the mixture models. When $M_i = R_i$ the missingness can be classified into patterns. Pattern mixture models are attractive because they are amenable to the plots displaying the observed data as in Figures 9.1 and 9.2. The strong assumptions center around the extrapolation of the curves past the time of dropout. When the trajectories are linear (Figure 9.1), it may be very reasonable to extend the slopes for patterns with at least two assessments. The slope for the pattern with only baseline data will require an additional assumption, possibly using the slope from the pattern with two assessments. But when the trajectories are nonlinear (Figure 9.2), it can be very difficult to identify a procedure even after the results are plotted. Prespecifying the methods for extrapolation is almost impossible. One strategy that is used is to pool the strata so that all the model parameters are estimable. Pauler et al. [30] illustrated this in a trial of patients with advanced stage colorectal cancer where they did not form the strata based on the patterns of observed data but on a combination of survival and completion of the last assessment. First, they defined two strata based on whether the patient survived to the end of the study (21 weeks), then they split the patients who survived 21 weeks based on whether they completed the last assessment. They assumed that the trajectory within each stratum was linear. The assumption is that the missing data are ignorable within each stratum. This implies that within the group of patients who did not survive 21 weeks, there are no systematic differences between those who died early versus later, and within those who survived, there are no differences between those who dropped out early versus later.

9.4.4.2 *Joint Models with Shared Parameters*

In this class of models, we are jointly estimating the longitudinal trajectories of the QOL outcomes with another process, typically time to dropout, disease progression, or survival. The underlying assumption is that the data are MAR, conditional on the time to the event. The concept is that the random effects of the model for the QOL outcomes are correlated with the time to the event. Specifically, the individuals who experience an earlier event will tend to start with lower QOL scores and will decline more rapidly. This is illustrated in Example 1 (Figure 9.1), where those with early dropout tend to have poorer QOL scores at baseline and decline more rapidly. When applied to this study, estimates of the decline over time roughly doubled in both treatment groups (Table 9.2). This illustrates the sensitivity of within-group estimates of change to the missing data, but relative stability of the differences between treatment groups when studying two active interventions with similar survival and toxicity.

The most critical characteristic for the implementation of these models is that there is a variation in the random effect, particularly associated with change over time. There are a wide variety of parametric and nonparametric models [33,34,38] that have been proposed. Vonesh et al. [39] extended the model by relaxing the assumptions of normality, allowing distributions of the random effects from the quadratic exponential family and event time models from accelerated failure time models (e.g., Weibull, exponential extreme values, and the piece-wise exponential model). Numerous investigators have joined proportional hazard models with the longitudinal models.

TABLE 9.2

Example 1 (NSCLC Trial): Joint Model for FACT-Lung TOI and Various Measures of the Time to Dropout (T^D). Parameter Estimates of Intercept (β_0), Slopes for Control Group (β_1) and Experimental Group (β_2), and the Difference in Slopes ($\beta_2 - \beta_1$)

Dropout Event	$\hat{\beta}_0$	$\hat{\beta}_1$	$\hat{\beta}_2$	$\hat{\beta}_2 - \hat{\beta}_1$
None (MLE)	65.9 (0.66)	−1.18 (0.29)	−0.58 (0.19)	0.60 (0.31)
ln(Survival)	65.7 (0.66)	−1.85 (0.30)	−1.43 (0.24)	0.47 (0.31)
Last assessment	66.1 (0.66)	−2.15 (0.39)	−1.53 (0.31)	0.62 (0.32)

Other extensions include multiple reasons for dropout [3,9] and the possibility that some subjects would not eventually experience the dropout event and could stay on the intervention indefinitely [3,22,41].

9.4.4.3 Multiple Imputation

As the software for multiple imputation (MI) has become extremely accessible, it is being proposed more often to address missing data issues. Most MI techniques assume that the missing data is MAR conditional on the variables included in the imputation procedure. If the imputation procedure only includes the available information that will be used in the analysis (previous assessments, treatment assignment, and baseline covariates), the results will be very similar to those obtained from the likelihood-based methods previously described. Thus, there is a danger of believing that any bias due to missing data has been eliminated, when in fact it has not. In the context of oncology trials, if surrogate measures for the QOL response were available and were incorporated into the imputation scheme, the missing data might be MAR conditional on those measures. However, those surrogate measures are typically both unmeasured and unknown, limiting the usefulness of MI techniques.

9.4.5 QOL After Death

One of the most controversial areas of research involving QOL is the analysis of trials with significant morbidity. The controversy occurs because of philosophical issues about imputing a value for measures of QOL or other patient-reported measures. What is often ignored is that even if explicit imputation is avoided, most methods of analysis implicitly impute a value. This is most obvious when using the EM algorithm for likelihood-based methods. In the E-step, the conditional expectations of the missing assessments given the observed data are used for computing the sufficient statistics. One class of measures referred to as patient preference or utility measures (e.g., EQ-5D or HUI) explicitly defines death as a value of zero. These measures are typically used in health economics (e.g., estimating quality-adjusted life years (QALYs)) but less often when comparison of treatment arms is of primary interest.

9.4.5.1 Analyses that Avoid Imputation

There are a limited number of approaches that avoid imputation and are primarily descriptive. The first is to examine the trajectory as a function of the time prior to death (Figure 9.3). This is useful when trying to determine if and when there are changes prior to death. For example, in the NSCLC trial patient, the decline in the FACT-TOI measure tends to be quite gradual until approximately a week before death. A second approach also relies on graphical presentation, where subjects are stratified by the time of death in a manner similar to Figures 9.1 or 9.2. While it is possible to construct

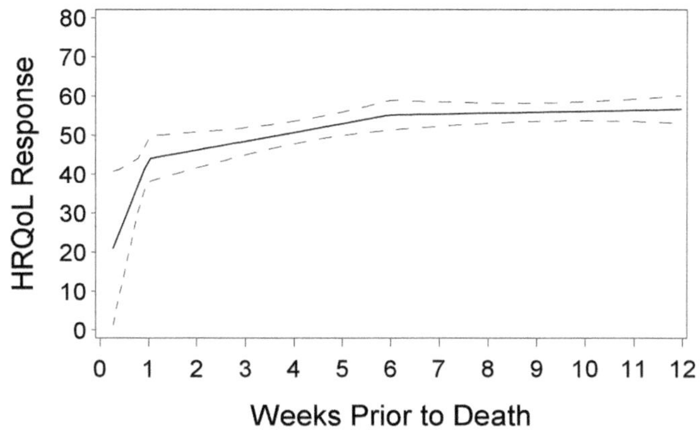

FIGURE 9.3
Estimated change in FACT-Lung TOI prior to death in NSCLC patients.

strata-specific contrasts of these trajectories across treatment groups [4], the interpretation is limited to just that and cannot be used as an overall comparison of the outcome under the intent-to-treat concept.

9.4.5.2 Explicit Imputation Methods

A number of simple imputation techniques have been described, but none have attained widespread use. An example of simple imputation is the substitution of an arbitrary low (or high) value for the assessments that occur after death [10,31]. Values of 0, as well as a value just below the minimum of all observed scores, has been suggested. Both approaches can be partially justified but neither can be completely defended. It also should be noted that when a large proportion of the subjects expire, the distribution of scores will tend to become bimodal, approximating a binary indicator for death, and the analysis becomes an approximation to the analysis of survival rather than QOL.

Diehr et al. [6] describe a variation on the last value carried forward procedure. In this procedure, a value δ is subtracted from (or added to) the last value observed. If this value can be justified, this approach could be a useful option in a sensitivity analysis. In Diehr's example, a value of 15 points on the SF-36 physical function scale was proposed, where 15 points was justified as the difference in scores between individuals reporting their health as unchanged vs. those reporting their health as worsening.

It is possible to utilize the MI methods in this setting. A variation of Diehr's approach could utilize multiple imputed values with varying values of δ as a sensitivity analysis to see if the results of treatment comparisons are robust to a range of values of δ. Alternatively, models similar to the one displayed in Figure 9.3 could be used as the basis for imputation of values at the time of death and beyond.

9.4.5.3 Implicit Imputation Methods

Joint models with shared parameters previously described in Section 9.4.4 comprise a wide class of models that can be used in trials with dropout due to death. As these are likelihood-based methods, they use implicit imputation of the missing data or the random effects in the estimation procedures, conditional on both the previously observed measures and the time to death.

9.4.6 QALYs and Q-TWiST

QALYs and Q-TWiST measures integrate quality and quantity of life; these measures may be useful when there are trade-offs associated with the interventions being assessed in the clinical trial. Questions of this nature are particularly relevant in diseases that have relatively short expected survival and the intent of treatment is palliative, such as in advanced-stage cancer. In contrast to the aforementioned analyses, in which the outcomes are expressed in the metric of the QOL scale, QALYs and Q-TWiST measures are expressed in the metric of time.

There are two approaches that might be encountered in a clinical trial. In the first, measures of patient preferences are measured repeatedly over time and the outcome is QALYs. In the second approach, the average time in various health states is measured and weighted using preference measures that are specific to each of the health states generating Q-TWiST estimates.

9.4.6.1 QALYs

In some trials, patient preferences are measured repeatedly over time, often using multi-attribute measures (e.g., HUI, EQ-5D, QWB) or transformations health status scales (e.g., SF-36) to utility measures [12,13]. The basis for all of the methods is an estimation of the AUC generated by plotting the utility measure versus time. There are two approaches. The first strategy estimates the average trajectory in each treatment group using a longitudinal model and then calculates AUC as a function of the parameter estimates in the same manner as described for health status measures. The difference is that since the preference measure is measured on a unit-less scale from 1 (perfect health) to 0 (death), the estimate can be interpreted as an estimate of QALYs.

The second strategy starts with the calculation of a value for each individual, $QALY_i$, which is a function of the utility scores and time. These values will then be subsequently analyzed as univariate measures. The calculation of $QALY_I$ depends on a rule for estimating the measure between assessments, possibly extrapolation back in time or using a trapezoidal function as illustrated in Figure 9.4.

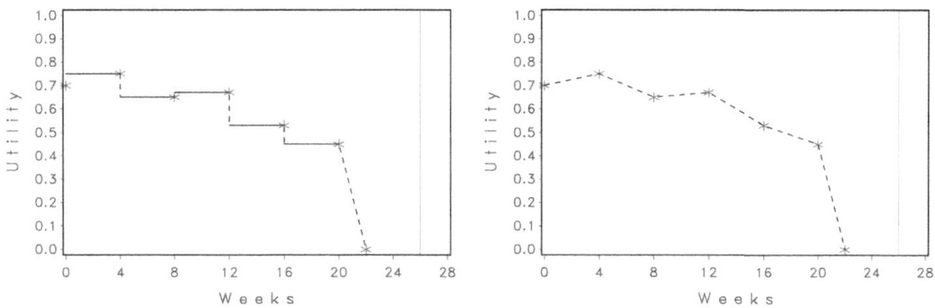

FIGURE 9.4
Illustration of two techniques to estimate $QALY_i$ when the time between assessments (4 weeks) equals the period of recall using horizontal (left) and trapezoidal (right) extrapolation. Observations are indicated by *. Periods using trapezoidal approximation are indicated by a dashed line.

The major limitation for both of these approaches is that all patients are rarely followed up until death and thus the estimates are limited to a fixed time period.

9.4.6.2 *Q-TWiST*

A second method used to integrate quality and quantity of life is Q-TWiST. A fundamental requirement for this approach is that distinct health states need to be defined. In the original application of this method [15] in breast cancer patients, four health states were defined:

TOX	the period during which the patients were receiving therapy and presumably experiencing toxicity;
TWiST	the period after therapy during which the patients were without symptoms of the disease or treatment;
REL	the period between relapse (recurrence of disease) and death;
DEATH	the period following death.

The second assumption is that each health state is associated with a weight or value of the health state relative to perfect health that is representative of the entire time the subject is in that health state. The assumption that the utility for each health state does not vary with time has been termed *utility independence* [15].

A third assumption is that there is a natural progression from one health state to another. In the above example, it was assumed that patients would progress from TOX to TWiST to REL to DEATH. The possibility of skipping health states, but not going backward, is allowed. Thus, a patient might progress from TOX directly to REL or DEATH, but not from TWiST back to TOX or REL back to TWiST. Obviously, exceptions could occur, and if very rare, they might be ignored. The quantity Q-TWiST is a weighted score of the average time spent in each of these health states, where the weights are based on preference scores. Typically, the weight for the period of time without symptoms U_{TWiST} is fixed at a value of 1 implying no loss of QALYs and for the period after death, U_{DEATH} is fixed at a value of 0. Thus, for this example, there are only two potentially unknown weights, U_{TOX} and U_{REL}.

$$\begin{aligned} Q-\text{TWiST} &= T_{\text{TOX}} * U_{\text{TOX}} + T_{\text{TWiST}} * \underbrace{U_{\text{TWiST}}}_{=1} \\ &+ {}_{\text{REL}} * U_{\text{REL}} + T_{\text{DEATH}} * \underbrace{U_{\text{DEATH}}}_{=0} \end{aligned} \tag{9.5}$$

If all of the patients in the study have been followed up to death, finding the average time in each health state is quite easy as the time for each is known for every patient. But when there is censoring, we need to use methods developed for survival analyses. Figure 9.5 illustrates the Kaplan–Meier estimates for the time to the end of treatment (TOX), the end of the disease-free survival (DFS), and the end of survival (SURV) for the patients an adjuvant breast cancer trial with up to 60 months of follow-up. The average time in TOX is equal to the AUC for the time to the end of treatment. The heath state TWiST is defined as the time between the end of TOX and DFS. The average time spent in TWiST is equal to the area between the two curves. Similarly, the health state REL is defined as the time between the end of DFS and SURV. The average time in REL is again the area between the curves. When the follow-up is incomplete, we must estimate restricted means that estimate the average times in each health state up to a set limit. At the first glance, it might appear that 60 months (five years) would be a good choice. However, for practical reasons related to the estimation of the variance of the estimates, it is more appropriate to pick a time where follow-up is complete for 50%–75% of the subjects who are still being followed.

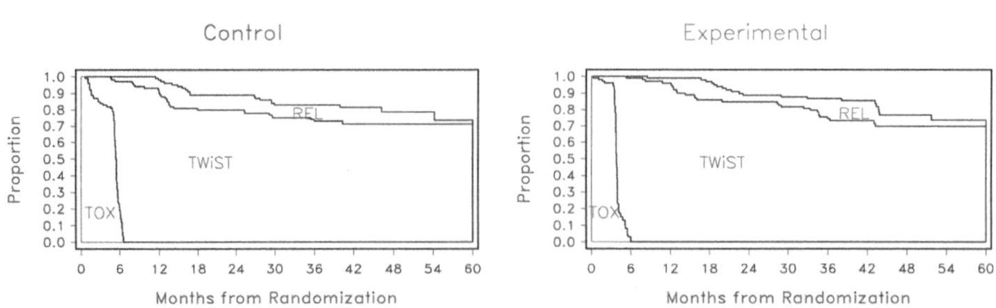

FIGURE 9.5
Partitioned survival plots for the control and experimental groups of the breast cancer trial. Each plot shows the estimated curves for TOX, DFS, and SURV. Areas between the curves correspond to the time spent in the TOX, TWiST, and REL health states.

9.5 Summary

Despite the challenges associated with the analysis of patient-reported outcomes in oncology trials, the results of these analyses are important to patients and care providers. The role of the statistician often goes just beyond the analysis plan. Often it is the statistician who is at the interface of the trial design and the analysis plan. It is in the development of an analysis plan that the goals of the trial as well as the specific aims need to be clarified. QOL and other patient-reported outcomes can provide useful clinical information; their role needs to be carefully and explicitly defined. The goals, the role, and the actual domains that are to be measured specifically influence the procedures that will be used to minimize the multiple comparisons as well as the strategies for missing data.

References

1. Bonomi P, Kim KM, Fairclough D, Cella D, Kugler J, Rowinsky E, Jiroutek M, Johnson D. (2000) Comparison of survival and quality of life in advanced non-small-cell lung cancer patients treated with two dose levels of paclitaxel combined with cisplatin versus etoposide-cisplatin: Results of an eastern cooperative group trial. *Journal of Clinical Oncology*, 18: 623–631.
2. Carpenter, JR, Kenward MG. (2008) Missing data in randomised controlled trials - a practical guide. Birmingham: National Institute for Health Research, Publication RM03/JH17/MK. Available at http://www.missingdata.org.uk.
3. Chi Y, Ibrahim JG. (2006) Joint models for multivariate longitudinal and multivariate survival data. *Biometrics*, 62: 432–445.
4. Dawson JD. (1994) Stratification of summary statistic tests according to missing data patterns. *Statistics in Medicine*, 13: 1853–1863.
5. Dempster AP, Laird NM, Rubin DB. (1977) Maximum likelihood estimation from incomplete data via the EM algorithm (with discussion). *Journal of the Royal Statistical Society, Series B*, 39: 1–38.
6. Diehr P, Patrick DL, Hedrick S, Rothaman M, Grembowski D, Raghunathan TI, Beresford S. (1995) Including deaths when measuring health status over time. *Medical Care*, 33(suppl): AS164–AS172.
7. Diggle PJ, Kenward MG. (1994) Informative dropout in longitudinal data analysis (with discussion). *Applied Statistics*, 43: 49–93.
8. Dmitrienko A, Offen W, Westfall PH. (2003) Gate-keeping strategies for clinical trials that do not require all primary effects to be significant. *Statistics in Medicine*, 22: 2387–2400.
9. Elashoff RM, Li G, Li N. (2007) An approach to joint analysis of longitudinal measurements and competing risks failure time data. *Statistics in Medicine*, 26: 2813–2835.

10. Fairclough DL, Fetting JH, Cella D, Wonson W, Moinpour C for the Eastern Cooperative Oncology Group. (1999) Quality of life and quality adjusted survival for breast cancer patients recieving adjuvant therapy. *Quality of Life Research*, 8: 723–731.
11. Fairclough, DL. (2010) *Design and Analysis of Quality of Life Studies in Clinical Trials*, 2nd edition. CRC Press, Boca Raton, FL.
12. Feeny D. (2005) Preference-based measures: Utility and quality-adjusted life years. In *Assessing Quality of Life in Clinical Trials*, 2nd edition. pp 405–429. Fayers P Hays R, eds. Oxford University Press.
13. Franks P, Lubetkin EI, Gold MR, Tancredi DJ. (2003) Mapping the SF-12 to preference-based instruments: Convergent validity in a low-income, minority population. *Medical Care*, 41: 1277–1283.
14. Freemantle N, Calvert M, Wood J, Eastangh J, Griffin C. (2003) Composite outcomes in randomized trials: Great precision but with greater uncertainty? *Journal of the American Medical Association*, 239: 2554–2559.
15. Glasziou PP, Simes RJ, Gelber RD. (1990) Quality adjusted survival analysis. *Statisitics in Medicine*, 9: 1259–1276.
16. Hicks JE, Lampert MH, Gerber LH, Glastein E, Danoff J. (1985) Functional outcome update in patients with soft tissue sarcoma undergoing wide local excision and radiation (Abstract). *Archives of Physical Medicine and Rehabilitation*, 66: 542–543.
17. Hochberg Y. (1988) A sharper Bonferroni procedure for multiple significance testing. *Biometrika*, 75: 800–803.
18. Hogan JW, Roy J, Korkontzelou C. (2004) Tutorial in biostatistics: Handling drop-out in longitudinal studies. *Statistics in Medicine*, 23: 1455–1497.
19. Holm S. (1979) A simple sequentially rejective multiple test procedure. *Scandinavian Journal of Statistics*, 6: 65–70.
20. Jennrich R, Schluchter M. (1986) Unbalanced repeated-measures models with structured covariance matrices. *Biometrics*, 42: 805–820.
21. Korn EL, O'Fallon J. (1990) *Statistical Considerations, Statistics Working Group. Quality of Life Assessment in Cancer Clinical Trials*, Report on Workshop on Quality of Life Research in Cancer Clinical Trials. Division of Cancer Prevention and Control, National Cancer Institute.
22. Law NJ, Taylor JMG, Sandler HM. (2002) The joint modeling of a longitudinal disease progression marker and the failure time process in the presence of cure. *Biostatistics*, 3: 547–563.
23. Little RJA. (1988) A test of missing completely at random for multivariate data with missing values. *Journal of the American Statistical Association*, 83: 1198–1202.
24. Little RJA. (1993) Pattern-mixture models for multivariate incomplete data. *Journal of the American Statistical Association*, 88: 125–134.
25. Little RJA. (1994) A class of pattern-mixture models for normal incomplete data. *Biometrika*, 81: 471–483.
26. Little RJA. (1995) Modeling the dropout mechanism in repeated-measures studies. *Journal of the American Statistical Association*, 90: 1112–1121.
27. Marcus R, Peritz E, Gabriel KR. (1976) On closed testing procedures with special reference to ordered analysis of variance. *Biometrika*, 63: 655–660.
28. Moinpour CM, Savage MJ, Troxel A, Lovato LC, Eisenberger M, Veith RW, Higgins B, Skeel R, Yee M, Blumenstein BA, Crawford ED, Meyskens FL. (1998) Quality of life in advanced prostate cancer: Results of a randomized therapeutic trial. *Journal of National Cancer Institute*, 90: 1537–1544.

29. Motzer RJ, Murphy BA, Bacik J, Schwartz LH, Nanus DM, Mariani T, Loehrer P, Wilding G, Fairclough DL, Cella D, Mazumdar M. (2000) Phase III trial of Interferon Alfa-2a with or without 13-*cis*-retinoic acid for patients with advanced renal cell carcinoma. *Journal of Clinical Oncology*, 18: 2972–2980.
30. Pauler DK, McCoy S, Moinpour C. (2003) Pattern mixture models for longitudinal quality of life studies in advanced stage disease. *Statistics in Medicine*, 22: 795–809.
31. Raboud JM, Singer J, Thorne A, Schechter MT, Shafran SD. (1998) Estimating the effect of treatment on quality of life in the presence of missing data due to dropout and death. *Quality of Life Research*, 7: 487–494.
32. Schafer JL, Graham JW. (2002) Missing data: Our view of the state of the art. *Psychological Methods*, 7: 147–177.
33. Ribaudo HJ, Thompson SG, Allen-Mersh TG. (2000) A joint analysis of quality of life and survival using a random-effect selection model. *Statistics in Medicine*, 19: 3237–3250.
34. Schluchter MD. (1992) Methods for the analysis of informatively censored longitudinal data. *Statistics in Medicine*, 11: 1861–1870.
35. Schumacher M, Olschewski M, Schulgen G. (1991) Assessment of quality of life in clinical trials. *Statistics in Medicine*, 10: 1915–1930.
36. Staquet M, Aaronson NK, Ahmedzai S, et al. (1992) Editorial: Health-related quality of life research. *Quality of Life Research*, 1: 3.
37. Sugarbaker PH, Barofsky I, Rosenberg SA, Gianola FJ. (1982) Quality of life assessment of patients in extremity sarcoma clinical trials. *Surgery*, 91: 17–23.
38. Touloumi G, Pocock SJ, Babiker AG, Daryshire JH. (1999) Estimation and comparison of rates of change in longitudinal studies with informative drop-outs. *Statistics in Medicine*, 18: 1215–1233.
39. Vonesh EF, Greene T, Schluchter MD. (2006) Shared parameter models for the joint analysis of longitudinal data and event times. *Statistics in Medicine*, 25: 143–163.
40. Wu MC, Bailey KR. (1989) Estimation and comparison of changes in the presence of informative right censoring: Conditional linear model. *Biometrics*, 45: 939–955.
41. Yu M, Law NJ, Taylor JMG, Sandler HM. (2004) Joint longitudinal-survival-cure models and their applications to prostate cancer. *Statistica Sinica*, 14: 835–862.

10

Impact of Evolving Regulatory Pathways on Statistical Considerations in Oncology Clinical Trials

Rajeshwari Sridhara

Center for Drug Evaluation and Research, U.S. Federal Drug Administration

CONTENTS

10.1 Introduction

There are two regulatory pathways for a product to be approved by the Food and Drug Administration for marketing in the United States. These are regular (i.e., full approval) and accelerated approvals. For regular approval, the product is required by law to demonstrate clinical benefit with respect to how long a patient is *alive, feels,* or *functions.* In the case of drugs for treating cancer, generally, clinical benefit is demonstrated in a randomized controlled clinical trial by comparing the experimental drug to a control, where the control may be a placebo, a best supportive care, or an active control treatment. By contrast, accelerated approval is based on a surrogate endpoint that is reasonably likely to predict clinical benefit for products developed for treating life-threatening diseases, and which demonstrate to be better than the available therapy. Accelerated approval is a conditional approval and products approved under the accelerated approval are required to demonstrate clinical benefit in the same or subsequent clinical trial(s). On the basis of the results of the confirmatory trial, a product first approved under accelerated approval is then granted regular approval if clinical benefit is demonstrated, failing which it is withdrawn from the market.

During different stages of the drug development, the manufacturing company or the sponsor of the drug product can apply for orphan drug, fast track, and breakthrough designations. The orphan drug designation is given to products that are being developed for use in orphan diseases with a disease prevalence of less than 200,000 patients per year in the United States. This designation provides an extended market exclusivity and waiver of the application review fee. A fast track designation is based on observed preclinical activity and allows for rolling submission of different sections of the marketing application. The breakthrough designation [1] (Food and Drug Safety Innovation Act 2012) allows FDA to expedite and assist drug manufacturers in the development and review of new drugs with preliminary clinical evidence that suggests that the drug may offer substantial improvement over available therapies for patients with serious or life-threatening diseases [2] (FDA guidance 2014).

During the course of drug development from very early stages to the approval of the product, statisticians play an important role in the design and conduct of the clinical trials and analyses and interpretation of the results. With the development of novel molecularly targeted therapies and immunotherapies to treat oncological and hematological malignancies, the demand from the patients and patient advocates for quicker access to new treatments along with the available newer regulatory tools, the complexity of the design, and analyses have become increasingly challenging. In this chapter, we will examine some of these challenges and how to address them.

10.2 Impact of Expedited Regulatory Programs

Pembrolizumab, an immunotherapeutic agent and PD-1 checkpoint inhibitor that has received breakthrough designation, was first approved under the accelerated approval regulations for the treatment of advanced melanoma, on the basis of the results from an expanded cohort of a Phase 1/2 study that included several cohorts with multiple diseases, multiple doses, and dosing regimens [3].

The decision of accelerated approval was based on a retrospectively selected group of patients with advanced melanoma who had received prior treatments, with an observed unprecedented durable response rate in this refractory disease where all patients had a minimum follow-up of 28 weeks. This Phase 1/2 study was first initiated as a single-arm dose-escalation study that included patients with advanced solid tumor malignancies. It was expanded to study the activity of the drug in melanoma and non–small cell lung cancer. Within each of these two diseases, several cohorts were expanded to evaluate different dosing regimens in refractory and relapsed settings with single-arm and randomized cohorts such that over 1,000 patients were eventually enrolled in the Phase 1/2 study. These expansions were based on accumulating data and observed results.

While expansions such as these are examples of the ways in which it is possible to accelerate drug development and conduct a study in an efficient, timely manner, they can result in a complex group of cohorts requiring careful planning, data collection, analyses, and dissemination to protect patient safety and address ethical concerns. First-in-human Phase 1 studies are exploratory studies to determine the optimal dose that can be safely administered in a large group of patients. As such, exposing large cohorts of patients to a drug for which there is limited safety information is detrimental to the public and drug development. However, for drugs showing high activity at the early development phase, it is paramount to consider different design options that would facilitate the rapid further development of the drug leading to market authorization and availability to the patients in need.

There are important statistical challenges in designing, conducting, analyzing, and interpreting the results in this type of expanded Phase 1/2 study. Among the questions that arise are the following:

- Are there prespecified objectives for each of the cohorts?
- Is there a potential for patient selection bias in these first-in-human studies?
- Can one aggregate data from different cohorts into one cohort to estimate an effect (e.g., objective response rate)?
- Is there bias in this aggregation and will the results be generalizable?
- Can different dose cohorts be combined together, assuming that the safety and activity are not different among the doses studied?
- Is there randomized allocation of treatments in some of the cohorts?
- Are the hypotheses prespecified along with the decision criteria consistent with the objectives of the study?

It is imperative to consider the objective and hypothesis for each expanded cohort in defining the starting and stopping criteria and the maximum sample size required to meet the objective of each of the expanded cohorts.

A key feature of these multiple-cohort expansion studies is that they have multiple objectives. It is critical that comprehensive data are collected and that the flow of data on safety and activity of the drug is seamless across the different cohorts in different diseases, so that the patients and the investigators are informed of safety concerns observed in other cohorts in a timely manner.

Such studies would greatly benefit from early planning, development of a master protocol with centralized operations and processes, and well-defined decision criteria for starting and stopping cohorts [4].

10.3 Impact of Molecularly Based Definitions of Diseases

With increased understanding of the molecular alterations underlying various cancers, it is becoming clear that within a category defined by histologic criteria, there are many distinct diseases with differing prognoses and responses to molecularly targeted therapies (non–small cell lung cancer is a case in point) [5]. The incidence of these molecularly defined diseases may be low and this will make it challenging to conduct trials of sufficient power. In this scenario, several options may be considered as listed here, although randomized trials are the preferred options even in rare diseases, provided they are ethical and feasible to conduct. For example, eculizumab was approved (regular approval) for the treatment of paroxysmal nocturnal hemoglobinuria based on demonstrated benefit from a randomized clinical trial comparing eculizumab (43 patients) to placebo (44 patients) [6].

I. *Randomized Clinical Trials*: Randomized clinical trials with unequal allocation such as a 2:1 or 3:1 randomization with fewer patients assigned to receive placebo, best supportive care, or standard of care can be considered. While they are not as efficient as those using a 1:1 design, in such trials, fewer patients are exposed to placebo or best supportive care, and therefore, they may be attractive to patients considering enrolling in a clinical trial. This would be a good design to evaluate both efficacy and safety. For example, siltuximab was approved (regular approval) for the treatment of Castleman's disease (prevalence < 1/100,000) based on a placebo-controlled, double-blind, randomized study with a 2:1 randomization allocation (53 patients: 26 patients) demonstrating a durable tumor and symptomatic response (34% response in siltuximab arm versus 0% in the placebo arm) [7].

II. *Single-arm Clinical Trials*: In a non-randomized single-arm clinical trial, it is assumed that zero or minimal response is expected when no treatment or placebo is administered. Although basal cell carcinoma is one of the most common cancers among Caucasians, metastatic basal cell carcinoma is rare, with a reported incidence of about 0.03% [8]. Vismodegib was approved (full approval) for the treatment of metastatic basal cell carcinoma based on a single-arm clinical trial [9]. In this option, while the activity of the product can be assessed, its long-term effect on time-to-event endpoints such as time to disease progression or overall survival cannot be evaluated due to confounding by the natural history of the disease. It is also not possible to conduct a comprehensive evaluation of safety as the association of toxicity with the drug can be confounded by the disease process. Only monotherapy can be evaluated in a single-arm study as the contribution of each of the components in a combination therapy cannot be assessed with this clinical trial design unless there is compelling external data regarding contribution of the components of the combination.

III. *Randomized Clinical Trial in Multiple Diseases*: A randomized clinical trial in which diseases that share, for example, a similar molecular pathway, and in which the difference between the experimental and control treatments is expected to be similar across these diseases can be another option. In this design, several rare diseases can be combined together using stratified randomization, if feasible, with each disease as a stratum. The conclusion regarding treatment effect will be applicable to all diseases included in the clinical trial. There is always a risk in assuming that the treatment effect would be the same or similar across all diseases, and given the rarity of the diseases and paucity of data, we may not be able to validate this assumption. If a registry is maintained for each of the rare diseases for tracking their natural history with sufficient follow-up and use of available treatments, then potentially such data could be used to justify a clinical trial of this type. This type of clinical trial design has been used in clinical trials evaluating chemotherapy, which includes all non–small cell lung cancer patients, irrespective of the histology and mutational status of the disease. More commonly, single-arm clinical trials with multiple cohorts of patients with different diseases and a common molecular pathway have been conducted [4]. For example, imatinib mesylate was evaluated for the treatment of 40 different rare diseases, all sharing a common molecular driver, BCRABL translocation [10].

IV. *Use of a Historical Control*: Historical control designs are usually reserved for special circumstances, such as when the disease has "high and predictable mortality (for example, certain malignancies) and studies in which the effect of the drug is self-evident (for example, general anesthetics...)" (21CFR 314.126) [11]. The ICH E10 guideline [12] also states that "the inability to control bias restricts the use of the external control design to situations in which the effect of treatment is dramatic and the usual course of the disease is highly predictable." For example, Vistogard was recently approved as the treatment for patients who received overdose or early onset of severe or life-threatening toxicities within 96h following the end of fluorouracil or capecitabine administration. In a retrospective analysis of historical case reports of 25 patients who were overdosed with fluorouracil and received supportive care, 84% died. On the other hand, only 4% of the 135 patients treated with Vistogard died in two prospectively conducted single-arm trials [13].

In a life-threatening rare disease where a randomized study is not feasible and the disease characteristics are well documented, use of a historical control with a prespecified process for collecting historical control information and a statistical analysis plan may be considered. There are different methods by which historical data can be used. One method is the use of propensity scores (PS) as a key design tool. The goal is to replicate a randomized experiment by forming groups with similar baseline covariates in the historical and clinical trial. Randomization ensures the balance of known and unknown baseline covariates between treatment arms so that any difference in outcome is attributable to the difference in treatment effect, and thus an unbiased estimate of the treatment effect can be obtained. In the absence of randomization, the idea is to have the historical control group and the experimental treatment group identical with respect to baseline covariates. Note that this is only possible for the covariates that have been observed and recorded. A PS characterizes the relationship between covariates and the treatment [14,15,16]. It is the conditional probability that a patient will receive a treatment (T) given the covariates (X), that is, $\text{PS} = P(T = 1 \mid X)$. PS is independent of the outcome (Y) and is used as a balancing score. If two patients have the same PS, then they have the same probability of receiving a treatment, thus mimicking a randomized trial. By matching patients in the historical control group and the experimental treatment group based on PS, one could compare the two groups to obtain an average treatment effect (ATE), that is, $\text{ATE} = E[Y(1) \mid \text{PS}] - E[Y(0) \mid \text{PS}]$. Note that there are other alternative approaches such as matched sampling and covariate-adjusted regression methods that can also be used sample size permitting [17,18]. The key assumption in these methods is that there is no bias in treatment assignment, that is, conditional on measured baseline covariates, the potential outcome is independent of treatment assignment. Additional assumptions include no unmeasured confounders, the probability of assigning a treatment not equal to zero, and treatment assignment of one patient not affecting the potential outcome of other patients. There are other challenges with respect to ensuring data quality (e.g., missing, inconsistent, or inaccurate data) and the historical control sample size (e.g., very large or very small, and difficult to verify if some patients were preferentially allocated to a treatment).

For a product to receive accelerated approval, there must be sufficient evidence that it is better than the available therapy. Often, this requires reviewing the literature reports on currently used or available therapy for that particular disease indication. For example, blinatumomab was approved under the accelerated approval regulation for the treatment of patients with Philadelphia chromosome–negative, relapsed or refractory, precursor B-cell acute lymphoblastic leukemia (B-cell ALL) (which is an uncommon form of ALL) based on a multicenter, single-arm study in 185 patients with the objective to demonstrate that the lower 95% confidence limit of the response rate is >30%. A response rate (complete remission or complete remission with partial hematological recovery) of 42% (95% CI: 34%, 49%) was observed in this study, satisfying the pre-specified objective criterion. In this example, to allow for a better understanding of the result in the context of the heterogeneity of the patient population with regard to prognostic factors, the sponsor provided a weighted analysis of patient-level data from 694 historical controls showing that the response rate was 24% (95% CI: 20%, 27%) in patients who had received available therapy. This confirmed that the target lower limit of 30% was reasonable and provided evidence that blinatumomab was better than the available therapy for accelerated approval consideration [19].

In a Phase II clinical trial with multiple cohorts of different diseases where a new treatment is being evaluated for all the diseases, a Bayesian hierarchical model that borrows information across patient groups has been proposed by Berry et al. [20]. This model inherently assumes that there is some commonality between individual cohorts of diseases with respect to the treatment effect on the disease, which allows borrowing of information such that the group-specific estimates of effect are "shrunk" toward the overall mean. The approach reduces the influence of outliers in the groups with very small sample sizes and results in more precise estimates of effect. Simon et al. [21] have proposed a Bayesian basket design with multiple strata of genomic variants within, for example, the same histologic type. In this design, a Bayesian approach is used with a two-point parameter space for each stratum similar to the commonly used optimal two-stage designs [22] by specifying too low or adequately high drug activity that would lead to termination or continuation of the further development of the drug. The decision to stop further development or to continue to develop further in a given strata is based on the posterior probability that depends on the numbers of responses and sample sizes in each of the strata at that time. This design allows for uncertainty regarding correlation among the stratum-specific drug activities and borrows across strata accordingly. Other Bayesian methods have also been proposed such as adaptive adjustment of the randomization ratio using historical control data [23]. In this method, an adaptive randomization procedure is implemented for allocating patients to the control arm aimed at balancing total information (concurrent and historical) among the study arms, and the idea is to assign more patients for receiving the experimental drug if the concurrent and historical controls are homogeneous. Balancing information as data accrues requires interim assessment of the relative informativeness of the historical data. Commensurate priors are utilized to assess the heterogeneity between historical and concurrent control and to borrow from historical data for the final analysis. A commensurate prior approach enables estimation of the extent to which corresponding parameters from different data sources have similar posteriors through the specification of a specific hierarchical model. Commensurate prior distributions average model parameters defined in the context of the likelihood for the current data at their historical counterparts [24]. Initially, patients are randomized 1:1 to the treatment and subsequently adaptively allocated based on an interim assessment of historical and concurrent control heterogeneity. The adaptation is based on the effective sample size that characterizes relative informativeness defined in the context of a piecewise exponential model for a time-to-event endpoint. If the accrual of patients is nonuniform and occurs in clusters, adaptive randomization could potentially lead to biased results and may also be difficult to apply when there is informative censoring in time-to-event analysis.

10.4 Summary

This chapter presents regulatory tools and pathways for seeking marketing approval of a drug product based on results from well-controlled and adequate clinical trials. New regulations make it possible to use tools that have the potential to accelerate drug development by taking advantage of the advances in understanding each disease at a molecular level. In this accelerated drug development time, it is important to consider carefully the clinical trial design options. While we have presented some design options, they are by no means exhaustive. The design selection should be based on the research question that needs to be answered and the feasibility of conducting the trial that would lead to a meaningful interpretation of the results. Electronic health record data from the real world to complement data obtained from clinical trials is an additional data source to be considered. The complexity of using such data is beyond the scope of this chapter.

References

1. Food and Drug Administration Safety and Innovation Act 2012. https:/www.gpo.gov/fdsys/pkg/BILLS-112s3187enr/pdf/BILLS-112s3187enr.pdf.
2. Guidance for Industry Expedited Programs for Serious Conditions – Drug and Biologics. 2014. http://www.fda.gov/downloads/Drugs/Guidances/UCM358301.pdf.
3. Khoja L, Butler M, Kang SP, Ebbinghaus S, Joshua AM. Pembrolizumab. *Journal of ImmunoTherapy of Cancer.* 2015; 3: 36.
4. Sridhara R, He K, Nie L, Shen YL, Tang S. Current statistical challenges in oncology clinical trials in the era of targeted therapy. *Statistics in Biopharmaceutical Research.* 2015; 7(4): 348–356.
5. Naidoo J, Drilon A. Molecular diagnostic testing in non-small cell lung cancer. *The American Journal of Hematology/Oncology.* 2014; 10: 4–11.
6. Eculizumab product label: http://www.accessdata.fda.gov/drugsatfda_docs/label/2017/125166s417lbl.pdf.
7. Siltuximab product label: http://www.accessdata.fda.gov/drugsatfda_docs/label/2014/125496s000lbl.pdf.
8. Uzquiano MC, Prieto VG, Nash JW, Ivan DS, Gong Y, Lazar AJF, Diwan AH. Metastatic basal cell carcinoma exhibits reduced actin expression. *Modern Pathology.* 2008; 21: 540–543.

9. Vismodegib product label: http://www.accessdata.fda.gov/drugsatfda_docs/label/2016/203388s010lbl.pdf.
10. Heinrich MC, Joensuu H, Demetri GD, Corless CL, Apperley J, Fletcher JA, Soulieres D, Dirnhofer S, Harlow A, Town A, McKinley A, Supple SG, Seymour J, DiScala L, Van Oosterom A, Herrmann R, Nikolova Z, McArthur AG, Imatinib Target Exploration Consortium Study B2225. Phase II, open- label study evaluating the activity of imatinib in treating life-threatening malignancies known to be associated with imatinib-sensitive tyrosine kinases. *Clinical Cancer Research*. 2008; 14: 2717–2725.
11. 21 Code of Federal Regulations Part 314.126.
12. ICH Harmonised Tripartite Guideline. Choice Of Control Group And Related Issues In Clinical Trials E10. 2000. https://www.ich.org/fileadmin/Public_Web_Site/ICH_Products/Guidelines/Efficacy/E10/Step4/E10_Guideline.pdfJournal>
13. Vistogard product label: http://www.accessdata.fda.gov/drugsatfda_docs/label/2015/208159s000lbl.pdf.
14. Rosenbaum PR, Rubin DB. The central role of the propensity score in observational studies for causal effects. *Biometrika*. 1983; 70: 41–55.
15. D'Agostino RB. Jr. Propensity score methods for bias reduction in the comparison of a treatment to a non-randomized control group. *Statistics in Medicine*. 1998; 17: 2265–2281.
16. Stuart EA. Matching methods for causal inference: A review and a look forward. *Statistical Science*. 2010; 25: 1–21.
17. Rubin DB. Using multivariate matched sampling and regression adjustment to control bias in observational studies. *Journal of American Statistical Association*. 1979; 74: 318–328.
18. Capeda MS, Boston R, Farrar JT, Strom BL. Comparison of logistic regression versus propensity sore when the number of events in low and there are multiple confounders. *American Journal of Epidemiology*. 2003; 158: 280–87.
19. Blinatumomab product label: http://www.accessdata.fda.gov/drugsatfda_docs/label/2016/125557s005s006lbl.pdf.
20. Berry SM, Broglio KR, Groshen S, Berry DA. Bayesian hierarchical modeling of patient subpopulations: Efficient designs of Phase II oncology clinical trials. *Clin Trials*. 2013; 10: 720–734.
21. Simon R, Geyer S, Subramanian J, Roychowdhury S. The Bayesian basket design for genomic variant-driven phase II trials. *Seminars in Oncology*. 2016; 43: 13–18.
22. Simon R. Optimal two-stage designs for phase II clinical trials. *Control Clin Trials*. 1989; 10: 1–10.
23. Hobbs BP, Carlin BP, Sargent DJ. Adaptive adjustment of the randomization ratio using historical control data. *Clin Trials*. 2013; 10: 430–440.
24. Hobbs BP, Sargent DJ, Carlin BP. Commensurate priors for incorporating historical information in clinical trials using general and generalized linear models. *Bayesian Analysis*. 2012; 7: 639–674.

Index

Q

T

U

V

W

For Product Safety Concerns and Information please contact our EU representative GPSR@taylorandfrancis.com Taylor & Francis Verlag GmbH, Kaufingerstraße 24, 80331 München, Germany

Batch number: 10725802

Printed by Printforce, the Netherlands